Intermittent Fasting & Keto Hacks

How To Turn Your Body Into A Fat-Burning Machine And Lose 20 Pounds In 30 Days!

By

Cameron Lambert

Table of Contents

Introduction **6**

Chapter 1: Intermittent Fasting In A Nutshell **10**

So, What Is So Good About Intermittent Fasting? 10

A Quick Summary 18

Chapter 2: Types Of Intermittent Fasting **19**

What Protocols Are Involved With Intermittent Fasting? 19

Our Focused Method 24

Chapter 3: The First Steps **25**

So, How Do You Get Started? 25

Hunger Vs. Appetite. What Is The Difference? 26

Not Great At Staying Hydrated? 28

Will Coffee-Drinkers Have To Give Up Their Delicious Coffee During Intermittent Fasting? 31

Make Sure You Are Also Getting Proper Sleep! ... 32

Be Careful When You Are Breaking Your Fast 33

Chapter 4: Stick To The Plan 37

How Do You Gain Success With Your New Routine? 37

What Happens If You Find Yourself At A Social Gathering With Food And You Are In Your Fasting Period? 42

A Few Points To Keep In Mind To Increase Your Success 43

What About If You Get Off Schedule? 47

Chapter 5: What Constitutes The Ketogenic Diet 49

Alright, So We Get What Intermittent Fasting Is. But Now What Is The Ketogenic Diet? 49

A Quick Summary 55

But What Should I Be Eating? 56

Chapter 6: Types Of Keto Diet 62

What Differs Between The Keto Diet Subtypes? .. 62

Chapter 7: Bringing It All Together 67

Firstly, Is It SAFE To Combine The Two? 67

Now, How Do You SUCCESSFULLY Combine The Two Methods? 69

Chapter 8: Making It Easy To Stick With It 71
    Having Trouble With Your New Eating Habits? ... 71

Chapter 9: Some Commonly Asked Questions 76

Chapter 10: Know Your Macros 88
    Let Us Use An Example 89

Chapter 11: Understanding Your Protein 93

Chapter 12: Speeding Things Up 96
    Let Us Start With Speeding Up Intermittent Fasting 96
    Now How About Enhancing The Keto Diet 99

Chapter 13: The Dangers Of Deficiency 104
    What Symptoms Should You Be Watching For? . 104

Chapter 14: Using Supplements 117
    Which Supplements Would Be Beneficial? 117

Chapter 15: Getting Active 123

Some Questions You May Have Surrounding Exercise With Intermittent Fasting 123
Let Us Look At A Few Facts About Exercising While On The Keto Diet 129
So, What Are Some Tricks To Maximize Your Results When You Are In Ketosis?....................... 132

Chapter 16: Keeping An Eye On The Calories 135

Chapter 17: An Example Routine 141
Here Is A List Of Healthy Keto-Friendly Meals To Break Your Fast With 146

Conclusion.. 152

References.. 156

Disclaimer 176

Introduction

Weight loss is something many people struggle with. The internet is full of different weight-loss strategies, all being shoved in our faces as the superior approaches. How do you know what is the best method? Which will give you the best results?

In this book, I am going to show you the benefits of combining intermittent fasting with the ketogenic diet for your weight loss journey.

Being in the field of health and well-being, it is important to us that we fully understand what we are promoting. The ultimate goal is to help our readers live healthier, happier lives – that is why we are in this field! Therefore, we have done the research, read through many different clinical trials to determine how and why these methods are so efficient. Backed by these scientific studies, intermittent fasting and the keto diet, separately, are effective in eliminating excess fat, reducing cholesterol, and improving overall health. Combine both methods, and you have an unstoppable strategy!

A healthier, happier life is something we all strive for! For those of you who struggle to lose that excess weight, following these dietary methods can not only help you achieve your goal, but you will not feel like you are overly restricting yourself in the process. You will not have to give up all your favorite dishes completely, and the types of food this diet focuses on are large in variety and full of flavor! Lovers of fine food will still be able to enjoy plenty of delicious meals. **Our promise to you** is through this book, you will be given the information and tools to help you succeed in losing weight and having a healthier lifestyle. What you are about to read will give you the breakdown of how intermittent fasting and the keto diet work and how to start them, and then expands on how to incorporate them together successfully. Later chapters also address common pitfalls and how to recover from them, as well as how to make sure your body is still getting all its needs met. Each chapter will provide you with more tools for your arsenal against excess body weight. **Just have a look at the following testimonials:**

"After 3 months on keto with intermittent fasting, even with slip-ups at times, I was able to lose 50lbs. Once my weight stabilized with going back to a regular diet, I found myself with a smaller appetite, greater energy, and the weight stayed off." – Byron P.

"When I started intermittent fasting and keto, it was very challenging to fight the cravings to snack during my fasting periods. After several days however, I no longer felt those cravings, and it became a habit. I have been doing both now for 2 months, and I've lost about 20 pounds. It has changed not only how I approach food, but my overall lifestyle. I have the energy and mental fortitude to pursue activities I've always wanted." – Eli H.

So why not start **RIGHT NOW**? With our tips and tricks, you can be well on your way down your weight loss journey towards a healthier you! Take a chance and dive in **TODAY**! The sooner you start, the sooner you will begin to see results. Before you know it, you will be a natural, slipping into this lifestyle as if you have been doing it all your life.

Chapter 1: Intermittent Fasting In A Nutshell

So, What Is So Good About Intermittent Fasting?

The key to intermittent fasting lies not in what you eat, but more so **when** you eat. It allows the body to use its own energy reserves during periods of fasting instead of restricting the types of food you eat. This method typically involves 1-3 days a week of restricted energy intake, during which the body experiences a decrease in fasting insulin to allow stored **carbohydrates**, **proteins,** and **fats** to be released to generate the **energy** needed for daily living activities. Not only do these reserves get used but this also causes an increase in insulin sensitivity, leading to more efficient storage of these molecules during periods of feeding when insulin levels are naturally increased [1].

A significant effect observed from intermittent fasting that makes it so effective is its ability to **"flip" the metabolic switch**. This flip refers to the body's switch from using glucose to fatty acid and ketones, forms of fats, as its energy source. This is called entering 'ketosis'. Once glycogen, the body's storage of glucose, is depleted after a significant amount of fasting, the body will switch to breaking down fats. Allowing the body to tap into its own **fat stores** for **energy** is what makes intermittent fasting so effective in **weight loss** [2].

Many studies have been done over the years showing the effectiveness of this method for individuals trying to lose weight. One such study evaluated the method of **alternate day fasting (ADF)**, a subclass of intermittent fasting, where the individual alternated between **"feed days"** and **"fast days"**. On "feed days", the individual **eats normally**, whereas on "fast days" they reduce their eating to **only 25% energy intake**. Fifteen individuals underwent ADF over 12 weeks, and the results were compared to fifteen individuals who ate normally. Overall results from the study showed promising outcomes as a weight loss plan.

Highlights of the results include:

- A **decrease** in **fat mass** (by 3.6 (±0.7) kg) and **triacylglycerol** (TG) concentrations (by 20 (±8)%)
  - Triglycerides are fat molecules found in your blood and stored in your fat cells
- An increase in low-density lipoprotein (LDL) particle size (by 4 (±1)) and plasma adiponectin (by 6 (±10) %)
  - LDL is considered the "bad" form of cholesterol, as a high amount leads to a buildup of cholesterol in your arteries. Small LDL particles have been linked to serious illnesses, while the larger ones are relatively benign.
  - Plasma adiponectin is involved in regulating glucose levels and fatty acid breakdown.

A major cause of the weight loss observed throughout the study was due to there being no increased eating on feed days, even after fasting, which lead to a higher overall energy restriction. Participants also experienced dietary satisfaction and increased feelings of fullness by the end of the study, likely contributing to adherence to this method [3].

Another study looked at how effective a **combination of ADF** and **exercise** was in terms of weight loss. Sixty-four participants were recruited and separated into four groups: **ADF + exercise**, **ADF only**, **exercise only**, and **neither**. The dietary component was divided into two periods, the first being a "fasting" period of only **25% energy intake over four weeks**, followed by a **normal eating period over eight weeks**. The exercise component involved moderately intense exercise. The combination group was determined to be preferable over the other groups, especially when examining **fat levels** and **body mass composition**.

For instance:

- Those in the **combination group** observed a **reduction** in **LDL** particles (by 12 (±5)%), an **increase** of **high-density of lipoproteins** (HDL) particles (by 18 (±9)%), and a **reduction** in **fat mass** and **waist circumference**.
- LDL was mentioned earlier as being the "bad" cholesterol. HDL, on the other hand, is the "good" cholesterol, bringing cholesterol from various parts of the body to the liver to be removed.
- An **increase** in **LDL particle size** was also observed in the **combination** and the **ADF only** groups (4±1 and 5±1, respectively).
- **Lean mass** was observed **to remain the same** in the combination group, suggesting only fat is being eliminated and not muscle [4].

A third study further showed the positive effects of **ADF** and how it **benefits non-obese people** as a model of dietary restriction. Sixteen participants were recruited and told to fast every other day over 22 days. Even though they all had **varying activity levels**, ranging from sedentary to very active, all observed **positive effects** from this method.

- **Weight loss** was around 2.5 (±0.5)% of initial body weight and 4 (±1)% of initial fat mass.
- **Fat oxidation increased** to ≥15 grams; however, there was no observed decrease in hunger on non-fasting days. The addition of a small meal on fasting days may aid with this.
- **Insulin levels** also **decreased** by 57 (±4)% during periods of fasting [5].
  - A lower level of insulin allows the body better access to its own energy reserves, facilitating weight loss and decreasing the feeling of hunger while fasting.

A fourth study compared the effectiveness of **intermittent fasting** against **on-demand intake** of a **very low-calorie diet (VLCD)** for maintenance of weight in **obese patients**. The study was conducted over two-years as a randomized controlled trial with 334 participants, each evaluated **over a 16-week period**. Every third month the intermittent group would have two weeks of VLCD, while the on-demand would only have VLCD when the bodyweight had passed the cut off level.

- The VLCD-based procedure proved quite effective regardless of the structure, showing a **weight loss** of 7 (±11) kg after the two years.
- Risk factors for cardiovascular disease **improved** as well, including **HDL, LDL,** and **insulin** [6].

A final study compared the effects of **intermittent energy restriction (IER)** vs. **continuous energy restriction (CER)** on weight loss and metabolic disease risk markers among a group of 107 overweight or obese premenopausal women. This study was conducted over **6 months**. The participants were randomly assorted into two groups, one including **25% energy restriction as IER** and the other, including **CER**.

The following results were observed:

- Both groups were **equally effective** for weight loss, where IER showed a mean weight loss of -6.4 (-7.9 to -4.8) kg vs. -5.6 (-6.9 to -4.4) kg for CER.
- Both groups showed a similar reduction in leptin, total and LDL cholesterol, triglycerides, and blood pressure.
- Although small, there was a **greater reduction** with **IER** for fasting insulin and insulin resistance. The observed difference between the two groups was -1.2 (-1.4 to -1.0) µU ml-1 for fasting insulin and -1.2 (-1.5 to -1.0) µU mmol-1l-1 for insulin resistance.

The results from this study suggest that using the IER method is just as effective in as CER in terms of weight loss and other health biomarkers, making it a potential alternative weight loss strategy that does not require you to completely reduce the amount of food you eat, just when you eat it. This makes it a better option for those who do not want to give up certain types of food that they love [7]!

A Quick Summary

Overall, these studies have shown the effectiveness of intermittent fasting in weight loss, as well as improving your health. The prolonged fasting depletes your body's storage of glucose, its primary source of energy. This causes a "flip" in metabolism from glucose-based to fat-based, resulting in an **increased breakdown** of your **fat mass** to be used for energy. The result is **weight loss**, as well as **regulation** of your **cholesterol** and **insulin** levels, making your body **healthier** and **happier**!

Chapter 2: Types Of Intermittent Fasting

What Protocols Are Involved With Intermittent Fasting?

Due to its increasing popularity over the years, multiple ways to do intermittent fasting have been developed. The effectiveness of each method is based on the individual doing it and their lifestyle. Listed below are the **top 7 intermittent fasting methods**:

12-Hour Fast

This method is a good beginner's option for those wanting to try intermittent fasting due to the shorter fasting period. The easiest way is to schedule your fast to include when you will be sleeping, for example, between 7 pm and 7 am. This will help the fasting period pass quicker, as you will be unconscious for most of it! Then during the day, you can consume your normal number of calories.

Some research has suggested that fasting between 10-16 hours encourages your body to switch to burning your fat stores for energy [8].

The 16/8 Method

This method involves fasting for 16 hours, and only eating during your 8-hour "eating window." During the eating period, the individual can fit 2-3 meals in. It is recommended for women to fast for only 14-15 hours, due to better results with a shorter fast.

Studies have shown how this method of fasting can boost metabolism, as well as increase weight loss efficiency [9].

The 5:2 Method

This method involves fasting for two days a week. The individual eats normally for 5 days a week while restricting to 600 calories on the remaining two days (500 calories for women). The fasting days are typically separated during the week. For example, people might fast on Monday and Thursday, and eat normally the other days. It is recommended to have at least 1 no-fasting day between the fasting days.

There is limited research on this method. A small-scale study looked at this fasting method in 23 overweight women. For the course of one month, the women were found to have lost 4.8% of their body weight and 8% of their total body fat. However, most of them returned to their previous measurements after 5 days of normal eating [10].

Eat-Stop-Eat

This method involves a 24-hour fast, once or twice a week. Individuals using this method tend to start with 14-16 hours and move up towards 24 hours instead of jumping straight to a full day. This type of fast can cause fatigue, headaches, and irritability. One important thing to note for this method is to eat normally during feeding periods, making sure to not gorge after breaking the fast. Many people will fast from breakfast to breakfast or lunch to lunch. They can still have water, tea, or other calorie-free drinks during the fasting period.

Research has shown that occasional 24-hour fasting can have positive effects on your health, including improving cardiovascular health [11].

Alternate-Day Fasting

This method was mentioned previously. It involves fasting every other day, by either not eating at all or only eating about 500 calories. Fasting an entire day might be a bit extreme for beginners, however, which is why it is recommended to eat a few 100 calories on fasting days when starting out.

Examples of the benefits of this method are discussed in chapter 1.

The Warrior Diet

This method involves fasting during a 20-hour fasting window and eating a huge meal at night. This eating window is typically only around 4 hours. Only small amounts of raw fruits and vegetables are allowed during the day, and then at night, there is a 4-hour feeding window to eat the one big meal. Food choices are similar to the paleo diet, which requires whole, unprocessed foods. These should include plenty of vegetables, proteins, healthy fats, and some carbohydrates.

One study that closely mimicked this method, including fasting for 20 hours, concluded that people who consumed meals over 4 hours in the evening had higher weight loss than those who consumed the same number of calories in meals throughout the day [12].

Spontaneous Meal Skipping

This method is another good type for beginners, as it involves skipping meals when it is convenient. This includes simply skipping meals when you are not hungry or too busy to cook and/or eat. As long as the actual meals involve healthy foods, this is an effective method. It may also feel more natural than other fasting methods [13, 14].

Our Focused Method

We will focus on the **16/8 method**! This method has shown to be relatively flexible and easily fit into many different lifestyles. On top of helping with weight loss, it has also shown to **improve blood sugar** (potentially decreasing the risk of diabetes), **boost brain function,** and **increase longevity** [1, 15].

Chapter 3: The First Steps

So, How Do You Get Started?

The first step is to determine **WHEN** your 8-10 hour feeding window will be. There a few things to consider when setting this time.

- Many people with busy lifestyles tend to skip breakfast due to lack of time; therefore, an appropriate feeding window for them would be from noon to 8-10 pm. This would allow for a healthy lunch and supper, with snacks in between. Fasting would occur overnight and in the morning.
- Other people prefer to eat breakfast, therefore if they start the day at 9 am, an appropriate feeding window would be 9 am to 5-7 pm. This allows for a proper breakfast and lunch with a snack right before starting to fast.

No matter when you start your fast, the important part is to **eat multiple small meals and snacks** spaced evenly throughout the day. This aids in stabilizing blood sugars and preventing spikes, as well as keeping your hunger from getting out of control.

Healthy Habits: sticking to nutritious foods and beverages can help maximize your health benefits from this fasting method. Important food groups to consider during your meals include **Fruits**, **Vegetables**, **Whole grains**, **healthy fats,** and a **source of protein**. Overeating junk food during your feeding windows could end up negating the benefits of the fast [16].

Hunger Vs. Appetite. What Is The Difference?

There is an important distinction between being hungry and having an appetite. The feeling of being 'hungry' is your body's normal sensation of having an empty/near empty digestive tract. This process is controlled partly by the hypothalamus, a structure in the brain, which has increased the firing of its neurons during periods of hunger [17]. Glucose and hormone levels, as well as how empty your stomach and intestines are, play a role as well [18]. Appetite, on the other hand, has to do with your desire to eat food. This can be increased by seeing, smelling, or thinking about food, whether hunger is present or not. Therefore, even if you are NOT hungry, your appetite may make you want to eat anyway [19]. During intermittent fasting, it is important to listen to your body during feeding periods, eating because you are **HUNGRY** not only because of an increased **APPETITE**.

Hydration is another important factor in this fasting method. Proper hydration is important for a variety of reasons.

- Balancing your acid-base levels
- Eliminating waste from your body
- Regulating hormone levels
- Transporting nutrients to the cells

On average, an individual should drink roughly 2L of

water each day to ensure proper hydration. During a fast, the body will lose a lot of fluid, causing an increased need for fluids. Therefore, it is vital to make sure you adequately compensate for this fluid loss. Calorie-free drinks like water, unsweetened tea and coffee help with hydration, as well as helping to control your appetite during the fast [20].

Not Great At Staying Hydrated?

Use an additive with your water. Not everyone likes the taste of plain water. Try adding a slice of orange or cucumber to it, or a leaf of mint to add some flavor. Some people even blend in a few wedges of watermelon.

Carry a water bottle with you. Easy access to refreshing water increases your likelihood of adequately hydrating yourself. Carrying a water bottle allows you to sip water throughout your day, guiding you towards your recommended hydration goal.

Create a hydration routine. Creating set times and intervals to drink water will help keep you hydrated. Phone alarms can be used to help you stay on schedule.

Try alternatives. While these options should only be used occasionally, alternating with the following can help make drinking fluids more interesting. Examples include:

– Tea
– Coconut water
– Electrolyte products

Eat plenty of raw fruits and veggies. These are loaded with water, making it easy for you to stay hydrated while also getting important nutrients. A few examples include:

– Berries (87-92% water)
– Baby carrots (87% water)
– Peppers (92% water)

- Celery (95% water)
- Cucumber (95% water)
- Melon (90% water)
- Spinach (92% water)
- Cauliflower (92% water)
- Tomatoes (94% water)
- Lettuce (96% water)

Soak chia seeds. These seeds can expand up to 10 times their original size when submerged in water, making them helpful in keeping you hydrated. Soaking them before consumption not only helps with hydration but prevents them from absorbing YOUR water, which would be counterproductive!

These options do not entirely replace drinking water! Regular water will always remain the healthiest option for you [21, 22].

Will Coffee-Drinkers Have To Give Up Their Delicious Coffee During Intermittent Fasting?

The short answer is: **NO**! But there is more to it than just that. Straight coffee has almost no calories; therefore, it will have a negligible impact on your calorie consumptions during the fast. It is when you start adding to your coffee (i.e., milk, sugar, etc.) that you start entering a grey zone, due to the increased calories.

Sticking with straight black coffee can actually have **benefits** during periods of fasting. Especially during the beginning stages of intermittent fasting, you may experience periods of mental and physical exhaustion as your body adapts to not obtaining energy from food. Having the caffeine can help you power through these difficult periods, keeping alert and focused enough to carry out your daily activities.

There is a **downside** to having coffee during your fast, however, and it has to do with resting. The fast allows your body systems to rest and recover, but coffee has awakening features, especially with your adrenal glands. These glands are involved with creating a stress response (your "fight or flight" instincts) by releasing a hormone called cortisol. Coffee could continually stimulate the adrenal glands to release cortisol, preventing the body from properly resting.

Is there a middle ground? Absolutely. While it is not recommended to drink lots of coffee during fasting periods, one or two cups will not undo the overall intermittent fasting benefits [23].

Make Sure You Are Also Getting Proper Sleep!

The best way to get through the physical exhaustion brought on by fasting is to make sure you are getting a decent amount of sleep at night. The recommended number of sleeping hours is between 7-9 hours each night [24], and when you are also running low on energy due to a reduced-calorie intake, those hours of sleep become even more important!

In fact, fasting before bedtime can indirectly help improve sleep quality. Studies have shown how nighttime eating can cause reduced sleep duration and quality, possibly due to the disruption of normal sleep patterns. Intermittent fasting prevents you from eating right before bed, helping to ensure you get a good night's rest. This, in turn, increases performance and concentration the following day, as well as vigor and emotional balance [25, 26, 27].

Be Careful When You Are Breaking Your Fast

One possible side effect of intermittent fasting is it could hurt your diet. A long period of fasting can build up your hunger, making you want to eat everything in sight when you finally allow yourself to indulge. This could result in overeating, however, especially if you are in a hurry to fill your empty belly. There is a relationship between the rate of eating and degree of satiation; if you eat quickly, you will consume more food before reaching satiety than if you eat at a slower rate [28]. This excess consumption could undo all the good you got from your fast, and even cause weight gain. Choosing to eat foods with empty calories will also negate intermittent fasting, even though your body will be craving sugary foods to replace its low blood sugars [29]. Having a plan in place when you break your fast will help keep you on track (i.e., appropriately sized pre-made healthy meals available, snacks are hidden away, or activities planned so that you will have to 'eat and go').

WHEN you break fast is also important to consider, as breaking fast at different times of the day have different effects on your body. The timing for starting and breaking your fast should align with your circadian rhythm. Our circadian clock has been linked to our metabolism, influencing our mitochondria function (the "powerhouse" of our cells), and the use of different fuel sources. Inopportune timing to break your fast could disrupt your sleep schedule, contributing to metabolic dysfunction, such as a decrease in growth hormone production and insulin sensitivity of your fat cells, and hampering your goals.

It may benefit you when starting intermittent fasting to track your blood sugar to determine and fasting schedule that works best for your body, in order to maximize your metabolic flexibility and health [30].

Important Tip:

Before you begin intermittent fasting for yourself, it is recommended you **talk to your doctor** to make sure it will be a good fit for you. This is especially important if you have **ANY** pre-existing medical conditions or you are taking **ANY** medications. In these cases, intermittent fasting could interfere and cause your body more harm than good.

IF YOU START TO FEEL SICK DURING YOUR FAST, THEN YOU SHOULD STOP. Take a step back and re-assess your plan. You can still achieve success with intermittent fasting, but you must make sure you and your body stay safe in the process!

Chapter 4: Stick To The Plan

How Do You Gain Success With Your New Routine?

So, you have got the basics, and you started implementing your intermittent fasting plan into your daily routine. The next step is to practice the method consistently. That means selecting your 8-8 hour feeding window and **sticking to** only eating in that period of time. This is the main way to achieve maximum benefits from intermittent fasting. The beginning stages will be tough, and you will likely be consumed by thoughts of food at the first belly rumble during the fasting window.

Therefore, during periods of fasting, it will be important for you to find ways to **KEEP YOURSELF BUSY!** The busier you are, the less time you have to focus on how hungry you are. Here are some ideas of how to distract yourself:

Drinking Water

The importance of staying hydrated was already explained in the previous chapter, but aside from keeping you healthy, it's the simplest and easiest way to stave off hunger. Very often, when you are feeling hungry, it is actually your body trying to tell you that you are thirsty. So, reach for your water bottle when you start feeling those hunger pangs!

Grab A Cup Of Tea Or Coffee

This is another hydration method that is a good option for suppressing hunger. Stimulating the nervous system and boosting your energy levels, tea and coffee options promote the feeling of being full. Caffeinated options also help keep you satisfied through a moderate influx of caffeine.

Get Your Chores Out Of The Way

Working on your household chores, such as cleaning or gardening, is a great way to distract yourself by shifting your focus. Not only will you be rewarded with a clean house and manicured yard, but you will also be able to grow your own delicious healthy food to eat when you break fast!

Be Productive

Think of all those tasks you have been putting off. Have a report to finish? Been neglecting your emails? This is the best time to get them done, as they will require your focus, keeping your attention OFF your hunger. Before you know it, it is time to eat!

Go For A Walk

Taking a brisk walk, like many other forms of exercise, can help keep your hunger levels down. It can be used as an enjoyable distraction while also supporting your overall wellbeing.

Play Some Sports

As mentioned earlier, physical activity helps suppress feelings of hunger. If you have a favorite physical hobby, such as tennis, basketball, or ultimate frisbee, jump into it during your fasting period. The fact that it will be enjoyable for you makes it that much easier to switch your focus away from your empty belly.

Engage In Short Bouts Of Intense Exercise

As it keeps coming up in this section, exercise should be one of your go-to's during the fasting period. Twenty to thirty minutes of intense exercises, such as weightlifting or sprinting, towards the end of the fasting period, is ideal. However, it should not be done every day (more on this in later chapters).

Meditation Will Help You Control Your Thinking

A more difficult method to use to suppress your hunger, but it is effective over time. With practice, you can get better at accepting and even embracing your hunger, while also controlling your stress.

Enter A "Controlled Fast"

If you have reached a point where you simply cannot control your hunger and NEED to eat something, choose to eat **lightly** through the fast. These include food that taxes your digestive system very little, such as live fruits and vegetables, which have the lowest glycemic index. Eating them in low quantities will help you make it through the fast when you are at your wits' end [31]!

It is also important to be aware of your environment. Where are your snacks stored at home? Keeping them out of view during the fasting periods will help you to control your hunger. As the saying goes, **"Out of sight, out of mind"**. The same goes for your work environment. Does your work have a break room? Is food generally visible? If this is the case, it is important for you to try to avoid those areas when you are still in the fasting period. Some ideas include taking a **different walking route** in your workspace that allows you to avoid the food area, or when taking your breaks **head outside for a quick walk**. Not only will being away from the food help with your feelings of hunger, but a little exercise will help increase your energy levels and control your food cravings. A study on rat models had even shown reduced consumption of food when exercise was combined with intermittent fasting [32].

What Happens If You Find Yourself At A Social Gathering With Food And You Are In Your Fasting Period?

Flexibility in intermittent fasting allows you to plan ahead for these events. If you have a friend's birthday dinner coming up end of the week, plan to skip breakfast that day so that you can shift your feeding window to include the evening. However, sometimes, social events arise spontaneously, preventing you from properly planning ahead. They are also much trickier to handle than your normal day-to-day life due to the unpredictability. Where will the food be (i.e., restaurant vs. dining room of someone's home)? What is being served? Can food be avoided?

The one plus of a social event is it is **SOCIAL**! You can distract yourself from food by socializing with the other partygoers (preferably away from the food). You can also do your best to make sure you are sufficiently full at the end of your feeding window, which can carry over to your fasting period and help keep the hunger at bay.

A Few Points To Keep In Mind To Increase Your Success

Approach Intermittent Fasting As If You Are Learning A New Habit

Most people are accustomed to the eating pattern of 3 meals a day, plus various snacks throughout the day. This standard eating pattern makes you feel like you SHOULD eat at a certain time (i.e., lunchtime), whether you are hungry or not. Starting intermittent fasting disrupts this pattern, making you consciously modify when you eat. Changing behavior is difficult, as it requires the input of a large amount of mental energy to keep it going. However, the continual practice of this new behavior will make it become a habit, and it will become a more natural eating pattern.

Be Strategic In Your Schedule But Remain Flexible

If your fast includes the morning hours after you wake up, you might need help getting through the "morning munchies" until you break fast in the afternoon. This requires planning ahead and making sure your last meal before starting the fast included balanced and satiating food, keeping you full for longer. However, if you are nearing the end of your fast, but you feel it is impossible to finish, it will not destroy all your progress if you break your fast early. You do not want to harm your body during the fast, and depending on how stressful your days have been, you may need that extra amount of food on one day to make it through your activities. Do not let it discourage you!

While it is important to plan ahead, at the same time,

remember that you should not allow yourself to overthink it! If you are too consumed with making sure you get the right amount of nutrition, it will be harder to keep your mind OFF food during the fasting hours. This will work against all that effort you put into keeping yourself full!

Get Pumped Up!

Intermittent fasting is a hard process to follow, but keeping a positive attitude can help you adapt to it easier. If you convince yourself you WANT to do it, then you will feel happier about sticking to it. It will be easier than trying to force yourself to do it. Try to focus on the positive side effects of intermittent fasting (such as weight loss, increased focus, etc.) to keep yourself motivated to succeed.

Keep Things In Perspective

Remember that fasting is not a new, unexplored process. You will always come across a new "lose weight fast" eating pattern, but fasting has been around for several years. It has been used for religious purposes, to make political statements, and to cure illnesses, among other reasons. If you know anyone who uses fasting for reasons other than weight loss, it might be encouraging for yourself to speak with them on their motivations.

Do Not Be Afraid To Fiddle With Your Schedule

You do not want the intermittent fasting process to feel like a form of punishment on yourself. If you feel that, for example, you will never be able to enjoy coffee again without a bit of stevia, add it! You do not want to create a negative relationship with food, where it makes you feel too guilty or restricted. There are no set rules for intermittent fasting, so feel free to play around with it to best suit your comfort level.

Also, do not be afraid to change the method you use for intermittent fasting as well. While this book focuses on the 16/8 method, a different method listed in Chapter

2 may work better for you. Do not be afraid to switch things up; it is important to find what works best for you [33]!

What About If You Get Off Schedule?

It happens! Even the best-prepared plans can be disrupted. Maybe those cookies your co-worker brought in were too tempting to resist while you were on your fast. We are all human – none of us perfect. The important thing is not to let it get you down. **One slip-up does not mean you should throw in the towel and give up on intermittent fasting.** Forgive yourself and get your schedule back on track, either picking up where you left off or starting over on Day 1. You could move your feeding window earlier in the day to include when you just ate and slowly move it back to where you originally had it. Or just keep it at this new time! Maybe this new time will suit your schedule better. The huge benefit of intermittent fasting is the flexibility it allows you, given you can set your feeding window at any time during the day, and how easily it is to move past small hiccups and successfully continue this method. **The important part is to keep at it!**

Chapter 5: What Constitutes The Ketogenic Diet

Alright, So We Get What Intermittent Fasting Is. But Now What Is The Ketogenic Diet?

Unlike with intermittent fasting, the ketogenic diet, or keto diet for short, regulates *what* you eat. The underlying mechanism of this diet is to change your body's metabolism from glucose-based substrates to ketone-based substrates [34]. This is done by implementing a **high-fat** and **low-carbohydrate** diet. Your body will first utilize the glucose you consume and deplete its reserves of glycogen for energy. However, due to the limited supply, this forces your body to **switch to fats**, or enter **ketosis**, to obtain its **energy requirements**. This results in **weight loss** as the body will now start to break down its fat reserves to be metabolized. This is similar to the effects of intermittent fasting, except it is caused by what you eat as opposed to when you eat. Another added benefit is the keto diet also **improves glucose tolerance**, allowing your body to regulate its blood sugars efficiently [35].

Like intermittent fasting, there have been many studies examining the effectiveness of the keto low-carbohydrate diet on weight loss. One such study compared the effectiveness of the **keto low-carbohydrate diet vs. low-fat, low-cholesterol, reduced-calorie diet**. The study recruited 120 overweight, hyperlipidemic individuals who were randomly assigned to receive the low-carbohydrate diet or the low-fat diet. The study lasted **over 6 months, with visits at 8, 16, and 24 weeks** to check various levels including serum lipids and other electrolyte levels.

- A larger number of participants in the low-carbohydrate group complete the study compared to the low-fat group, likely due to easier adherence to the diet restrictions (76% vs. 57%).

- After 24 weeks, there was a **greater weight loss** observed in the **low-carbohydrate group** than in the low-fat group (-12.9% vs. -6.7%).
- Those in the **low-carbohydrate group** also experienced a **greater decrease** in **serum triglyceride levels** (-0.84 mmol/L vs. -0.31 mmol/L) and a **greater increase** in **HDL** (0.14 mmol/L vs. -0.04 mmol/L) than those in the low-fat group [36].

Another study used similar parameters to examine the effect of a **low-carbohydrate diet** vs. a **low-fat diet** on weight loss and serum lipid levels in overweight adolescents. 16 participants were randomly assorted into the low-carbohydrate group, and 14 into the low-fat group. The study was run over **12 weeks**.

The following results were observed:
- This study also showed a **greater weight loss,** as observed in the **low-carbohydrate group** than in the low-fat (9.9 (±9.3) kg vs. 4.1 (±4.9) kg).

- There was also an improvement in **non-HDL cholesterol levels** (except LDL) in the **low-carbohydrate group** [37].

A third study compared the effectiveness of the **low-carbohydrate diet** on **weight loss** in individuals **with diabetes vs. without diabetes**, as most studies only consider individuals without. Thirteen individuals with type 2 diabetes and thirteen without were recruited and were randomly assorted into either a **low-carbohydrate diet group** or a **healthy-eating diet group**. The measured outcomes were weight loss, glycated hemoglobin (HbA(1c)), ketone, and lipid levels. The study lasted **over 3 months**.

- While no difference in HbA(1c), ketone, or lipid levels were observed (possibly due to the shorter length of this study compared to the previous one), there was a **greater observed weight loss** in the **low-carbohydrate group** (6.9 kg vs. 2.1 kg).

These results imply the diet is equally effective in individuals with or without diabetes [38].

A fourth study compared the **low-carbohydrate diet** against the **conventional low-calorie diet** and its **efficacy with treating obesity**. They recruited 63 obese individuals and randomly assigned them to the low-carbohydrate group or conventional group. The study was recruited **over one year,** and **measurements were taken at 3, 6, and 12 months.**

- Over the first 3 months, individuals in the **low-carbohydrate group** had **greater weight loss** than those in the conventional group (-6.8 (±5)% vs. -2.7 (±3.7)% of body weight).
- The **same** was observed **after 6 months** (-7.0 (±6.5)% vs. -3.2 (±5.6)% of body weight).
- There was **no significant difference** observed **after 12 months** (-4.4 (±6.7)% vs. -2.5 (±6.3)% of body weight).

- There was a greater increase in HDL concentrations and a greater decrease in triglyceride concentrations observed in the low-carbohydrate group throughout most of the study [39].

A final study examined only the **low-carbohydrate diet** and its efficacy in **treating morbidly obese adolescents** who weighed over 200% of the ideal body weight. Six morbidly obese adolescents were put on the **keto for 8 weeks**. This was followed **by 12 weeks of the keto diet plus two carbohydrates** (30 g) per meal (keto + 2 diet).

- Participants **lost** 15.4 (±1.4) kg during the 8 weeks of the keto diet, and an additional 2.3 (±2.9) kg during the keto + 2 diet.
- **Body mass index decreased** to 5.6 (±0.6) kg/m2 during the keto diet and an addition 1.1 (±1.1) kg/m2 during the keto + 2 diet.

- **Body fat** was shown to be **reduced** from 51.1 (±2.1)% to 44.2 (±2.9)% during the keto diet, and then to 41.6 (±4.5)% during the keto + 2 diet.
- **Serum cholesterol decreased** from 162 (±12) mg/dL to 121 (±8) mg/dL in the first 4 weeks of the keto diet [40].

A Quick Summary

Overall, these studies have shown the effectiveness of the keto diet in weight loss, as well as improving your health. By having a low-carbohydrate diet, the body is depleted of its primary source of energy, glucose, very quickly. This causes a "flip" in metabolism from glucose-based to fat-based, starting initially with the use of your dietary fat for energy, and eventually resulting in an **increased breakdown** of your **fat mass** to be used for energy. The result is **weight loss**, as well as **regulation** of your **cholesterol** and **glucose tolerance**, making your body **healthier** and **happier**! You may notice a similarity with the effects of intermittent fasting, mentioned previously.

But What Should I Be Eating?

The aim of the game in this diet is to lower your intake of carbs. Here are some examples of food groups you should focus on to ensure you also get your nutrients, which also have added health benefits [41]:

Seafood

Fish and shellfish contain essentially no carbs and have several vitamins, minerals, and omega 3. Fish intake has also been linked to a decrease in the risk of disease and improved mental health [42].

Low-Carb Vegetables

You will want to avoid the vegetables containing a lot of starch, such as potatoes, yams, and beets. Instead, focus on vegetables such as spinach, cauliflower, broccoli, and squash. Not only are they lesser in carbs, but they are also nutritious and could help decrease the risk of certain diseases [43].

Cheese

Both low in carbs and high in fat, cheese fits in well with this type of diet. It also contains lots of protein, calcium, and good fatty acids. One such fatty acid, conjugated linoleic acid, has been linked to fat loss [44].

Avocados

These are very healthy, containing lots of fiber and nutrients. They have also been shown to decrease LDL and triglycerides and increase HDL [45].

Fresh Meat And Poultry

These options contain no carbs and are a great source of protein and several nutrients, including B vitamins. The high-quality protein can help to preserve muscle mass [46].

Eggs

One of the healthiest options. With very few carbs,

eggs also have been shown to trigger hormones increasing feelings of fullness and keeping blood sugar levels stable, which decreases calorie intake [47].

Coconut Oil

This oil is unique in its composition. For instance, it contains medium-chain triglycerides, which can be converted to ketones or used immediately as an energy source. It has also been shown to promote weight loss and belly fat by increasing the metabolic rate [48].

Plain Greek Yogurt And Cottage Cheese

These options are both healthy and full of protein, although they do contain some carbs. They have also been shown to decrease appetite and promote fullness [49].

Olive Oil

While this oil contains no carbs, it has also been shown to decrease your risk for heart disease [50].

Nuts And Seeds

A high-fat, low-carb food option. They are high in fiber, helping increase the feeling of fullness and reducing the risk for different diseases (ex. heart disease, certain cancer, and other diseases) [51].

Berries

Unlike most other fruits, berries are low-carb and high in fiber. The antioxidants also aid in reducing inflammation and protecting against many illnesses [52].

Butter And Cream

While being nearly carb-free, it has been suggested that eating butter/cream in moderation may reduce the risk of stroke and heart attack [53].

Shirataki Noodles

This type of low-carb noodle is made of a viscous fiber,

which slows movement through the digestive tract. This helps increase fullness and regulate blood sugars, helping with weight loss and management of diabetes [54].

Olives

Like olive oil mentioned above, olives can decrease the risk of heart disease and potentially prevent bone loss [55].

Unsweetened Coffee And Tea

These drinks on their own are very healthy and contain no carbs. Not only can they boost your metabolism but have been shown to reduce your risk of diabetes as well [56].

Dark Chocolate And Cocoa Powder

This is a low-carb treat high in antioxidants, which may reduce the risk of heart disease [57]. Also, important to remember that the higher the percentage of cocoa it contains, the lower the number of carbs.

Chapter 6: Types Of Keto Diet

What Differs Between The Keto Diet Subtypes?

The ketogenic diet has also become a popular weight-loss method recently. This has led to a few varieties in the diet, which differ depending on your lifestyle. However, they all lead to the same end result, which is to bring you into a state of ketosis. Listed below are **4 variations of the keto diet**:

The Standard Ketogenic Diet:

This is the most common version of the keto diet. It is recommended for beginners, anyone who wants to lose body fat, and individuals with insulin resistance. In terms of your macros, your intake will look similar to this:

- Adequate protein intake (0.8 grams of protein per pound of lean body mass)
- 20-50 grams of carbs per day, or less than 5% of total calories

– A large amount of fat intake, or between 70-75% of total calories

The High Protein Ketogenic Diet:

This variation is similar to the standard keto diet, but with additional grams of protein. The purpose is to consume extra protein that can be used to build muscle. This makes it a popular method for bodybuilders, weightlifters, or those who need extra protein in their diet. On the high protein keto diet, your macro-level intake should resemble this:

– Fat is 60% of total calories
– Protein is 35% of total calories
– Carbs are 5% of total calories

Myth: Too much protein on the keto diet will kick you out of ketosis due to increasing gluconeogenesis (generation of glucose from non-carbs).

This is not true! The rate of gluconeogenesis is not the same as the rate of carbohydrate metabolism, which is the generation of glucose from carbs. Gluconeogenesis is a very stable process and will not result in a blood glucose spike when you eat extra protein.

The Cyclic Ketogenic Diet:

This method involves eating a low-carb keto diet for several days, followed by one to two days of eating a high-carb diet. Essentially, you are alternating between the two phases: a standard ketogenic diet phase followed by a carb-loading phase. This type is best for bodybuilders and other athletes to help maximize fat loss and build lean mass simultaneously. During the carb-loading phase, you will be getting roughly 70% of your calories from carbohydrates.

A weekly diet will resemble this:
– Five days of the standard keto diet:
    – 70-75% of calories from fat

- 20-25% of calories from protein
- 5% of calories from carbs
- Two days of carb-loading:
    - 70% of calories from carbs
    - 20-25% of calories from protein
    - 5%-10% of calories from fat

The Targeted Ketogenic Diet:

This type targets your carbohydrate consumption around your workouts. It is ideal to maintain exercise performance while fueling your muscles with glycogen. On this variation of the keto diet, you should aim to consume 25-30 grams of net cars roughly 30 minutes to an hour before exercising. This essentially covers your total carb intake for the day. This type is a hybrid between the standard ketogenic diet and the cyclical ketogenic diet. It allows you to train higher intensities at the gym without forcing you out of ketosis for extended periods of time (as would happen in the cyclic keto diet).

Our Focused Method

We will focus on the **Standard Ketogenic Diet**! This variation of the keto diet is the best method for beginners to start with, as it is the easiest to follow and keeps your body in a state of ketosis. It is the ideal method for those just looking to lose weight or have pre-existing insulin resistance [58].

Chapter 7: Bringing It All Together

So now that you have got the basics covered, where do you go from here? The next step will be to **COMBINE** the two weight loss methods. Overall, both function to "flip" that metabolic switch to start burning your fat for energy, meaning together they must make an effective team! Time to start examining how to incorporate both into your life.

Firstly, Is It SAFE To Combine The Two?

The short answer is **YES**! These two methods can essentially go hand-in-hand, as they tend to enhance one another and increase each other's benefits. Here are some of the reasons they make a great combination:

Enter Ketosis Quicker

The main goal of each is to bring you into a state of ketosis, burning your fat for your daily energy needs.

Having a keto diet causes your body to adapt to fasting with ketones, which in turn makes intermittent fasting more doable and easier to maintain.

Easier On Your Body

If you are eating a regular diet when doing intermittent fasting, the constant switching from glucose-based energy when feeding to ketone-based energy when fasting can cause great discomfort. Being on the keto diet keeps your body running on ketones, reducing that discomfort.

Lose Weight Faster

The keto diet and intermittent fasting complement each other well. People have generally been shown to naturally eat less often on the keto diet due to a higher level of satiety. This is handy when doing intermittent fasting because you will already be used to a larger period of time without food. As well, the smaller eating window helps to eliminate unnecessary snacking.

Stabilizing Blood Sugars

Continually alternating from glucose-based energy to ketone-based energy can lead to spikes in blood sugars, which can have negative side effects such as low energy and mood swings. Having a standard diet while doing intermittent fasting could cause these side effects, but being on the keto diet would completely eliminate them from happening [59, 60].

Now, How Do You SUCCESSFULLY Combine The Two Methods?

Here are 2 important tips to help optimize your efforts:

Ensure You Eat Enough

While you will be less hungry, it is still vital to make sure you are getting nutritious foods so that you will not develop any vitamin/mineral/etc. deficiencies.

A good list of nutritious ketogenic foods is listed in the previous chapter.

Keep Tabs On Your Ketone Levels

You can eat a certain amount of carbs while on the keto diet/doing intermittent fasting, but you want to make sure you do not eat too much that you kick yourself out about ketosis. **REMEMBER** that staying in a state of ketosis is how this process works and contributes to weight loss [59]!

Chapter 8: Making It Easy To Stick With It

Having Trouble With Your New Eating Habits?

Sticking to a new diet plan can be challenging for anyone, be it what you eat, when you eat, or both. The trick, as described by Dr. Eric Berg [61], is to determine what is specifically "throwing" your attempts and address them. A few examples include the following:

"I miss eating bread."

Easy fix. Do a quick google search on recipes on alternative bread that fit the diet.

"I feel so hungry!"

As mentioned before, your body will adapt to the new diet, and your hunger will decrease. It takes about 3-7 days for a noticeable difference, so just keep pushing!

"I am having trouble with the scheduling."

That is the great part of intermittent fasting. You can have set your feeding period at any time during the day! It lets you be flexible so you can still have meals with your family, make it to work commitments, etc.

"I feel deprived of my favorite carbs."

This can be addressed with some creativity, as other foods mimic carbohydrates (ex. potatoes, bread, etc.). Some examples include swapping:

- Tortilla wraps to lettuce wraps
- Hamburger buns to avocado halves
- Regular pasta to zucchini noodles
- Mashed potatoes to mashed cauliflower
- Potato chips to baked cheese chips
- French fries to zucchini fries
- Breadcrumbs to almond flour [62]

"I am bored with eating the same thing over and over."

There are so many options out there! Recipes upon recipes of keto-friendly meals. A quick google search or looking up some recipe books from amazon can help stave off the boredom and make your meals more interesting.

"This diet seems expensive."

In reality, it is quite the opposite. Intermittent fasting will limit your feeding windows, and the keto diet will naturally lower your appetite, both decreasing the amount of food you will consume and also decreasing your grocery bills.

"I am not a fan of salads."

Unfortunately, this barrier is unavoidable and needs to be overcome. However, by slowly bringing it into your diet, be it by having small servings or blending greens in your smoothies, as you start feeling healthier, you will likely become more receptive to having salads due to their positive impact.

"I do not like the side effects."

This diet can, unfortunately, come with a few side effects, including keto flu, keto rash, and fatigue. These can more or less be avoided if you are well prepared for the diet **BEFORE** you start it! Make sure you know the changes that you will experience and be ready to address them. This includes making sure you do not get vitamin deficiencies, making sure you get enough water, etc. Being properly prepared will help this diet be the most successful.

"The diet seems too restrictive."

The diet is only restrictive in terms of carbs and refined sugars. What you need to remember is there are so many alternatives (refer back to the earlier point)! It is also important to remember that these restrictions are what makes this diet so effective and working with them and finding alternatives that you are happy with are what will bring you success.

"The diet seems confusing."

When researching the diet, try not to use too many sources that may have conflicting information. Multiple sources of information can confuse you more than help, as different people will always have differing opinions on how to best approach the diet. It is important to find one solid plan and stick to that instead of trying to combine multiple plans.

"I am skeptical if this will work."

This is understandable. There are a lot of diet plans out there, and not all of them work. So why should this one? The best suggestion to get rid of your skepticism is to **TRY IT**. Plenty of studies have shown the effectiveness of this diet, meaning there is a high chance it should work well for you as well!

One final point to touch on in this chapter is instead of focusing on **weight loss**, focus on **getting healthy**! By eating properly and striving to maintain your body's health, this will naturally cause healthy weight loss and make you feel happier overall [61].

Chapter 9: Some Commonly Asked Questions

"How do you know when your body is in ketosis?"

Some signs that will point to your entering a state of ketosis include **decreased appetite, increased energy level, increased thirst and urination**, **"keto breath"** (fruity smell like nail polish), and **dry mouth** (or a metallic taste in your mouth). You can measure your ketone levels using urine strips, a breathalyzer, or blood meters.

"Can I chew gum on the keto diet?"

Yes, it is fine to chew gum on this diet, as the effects it would have on your diet is minimal. However, it is recommended to chew **xylitol gum** instead of those containing aspartame.

"Can I drink lemon?"

Absolutely! Lemon juice is not a big factor and is so

tart that it does not contain a lot of sugar.

"What about wheatgrass powder?"

Not a problem to have, even during the fast period. A good source of vitamins and minerals as well.

"Protein powder?"

This is fine to have ONLY during the feeding period, of course. Especially if it is whey or low-fat protein, it will spike your insulin, so you will want to add some fat to it and have it during or after your meal. This would not be suitable as a snack.

"Am I allowed cheat days?"

To get the most success from this diet, there are no "cheat days." The goal to keep your body in a state of ketosis so that it will effectively burn your fat away. If you "cheat" one day and eat a lot of carbs, you will bump yourself out of ketosis and have to do more work to bring yourself back to that fat-burning state. It could even take up to a week, so it is definitely not worth it!

"How do I make sure I am getting all my daily calories in one/two meals?"

The goal here is to avoid stuffing yourself and to make sure what you do eat is filled with lots of nutrients. Examples include **salmon over chicken** or **kale over other greens**. By having nutrient-dense meals as opposed to meals with empty calories, you will feel full faster, and your body will adapt to this method of eating less frequently. This will also prevent your metabolism from slowing down.

"How do I avoid getting a keto rash?"

This side effect can be caused by toxins in the body. Toxins are stored in the fat, and because you are burning your fat away, the toxins can come out and get into your circulation, causing a rash. This can be offset by eating a large number of vegetables, and also bentonite clay. The latter can be consumed on an empty stomach and is very effective at absorbing toxins in the body.

"What about an apple cider, vinegar, and lemon drink?"

No problem! These are acceptable to have even when on a fast period.

"What will happen to my cholesterol?"

For some people, there is a chance it can go up. This will especially be seen in individuals who are losing **A LOT** of weight. The reason for this is our fat cells are made up of stored cholesterol and triglycerides. When you are burning fat, your body is using the stored triglycerides for fuel, but the cholesterol is released as well. Due to this release, your cholesterol levels may go up. However, this is not something you should be concerned about because, for the vast majority of people, this excess cholesterol will be brought through the liver and broken down in the gallbladder for other uses.

However, it is also important to note that a small number of individuals may end up with continuously high amounts of total cholesterol. If you are concerned about your cholesterol levels on the keto diet, there are a few things to consider:

- **Stop drinking Bulletproof coffee**. If you eliminate significant amounts of saturated fat when you are not hungry, this may normalize your levels on its own.
- **Only eat when hungry**. This is where combining intermittent fasting with the keto diet can come in handy, as it might reduce cholesterol levels in some cases.
- **Consider using more unsaturated fats**. These include olive oil, fatty fish, and avocados. They will most likely help to lower your cholesterol.

If none of these steps help and your cholesterol is still abnormally high, consider whether you really need to be on a strict keto diet. If a more moderate or liberal diet can work for you, such as consuming 50-100 grams of carbs per day, it may help to lower your cholesterol. In these cases, you just need to remember to choose good unprocessed foods with high-fiber carbs, such as vegetables, nuts, and seeds, rather than wheat flour or refined sugar. **Consult with your doctor** if you feel medication therapy may be necessary.

"What can I do to avoid the keto flu/fatigue?"

This occurs when you are depleting your potassium and B vitamin levels. This is why it is so important to ensure you are maintaining your nutrient levels; keeping your potassium and B vitamin levels in the normal range will prevent this effect.

"Is this diet recommended when breastfeeding?"

Not really. This would not be the time to be concerned about your weight, as you want to ensure you are getting all the required nutrients so that you can pass it on to your baby. If you have a deficiency, your baby could as well.

"What about during pregnancy?"

No, and the reason is the same as for breastfeeding above. Just make sure you are eating healthy.

"Can children go on this diet?"

This depends. If the child is overweight, going on this diet should be fine. If they are not, however, they should go on a modified version of this diet that includes fruits, such as berries and bananas, and sweet potatoes, and yams. The difference with children is they have a very high metabolism compared to adults, so they will require some form of starch; otherwise, they will get too thin.

"Can I have Bulletproof coffee?"

The results with including Bulletproof coffee can vary from person to person. Some people have it in the morning and have it not affect them, but it has the potential to increase your insulin levels a bit, especially if you are adding fat or coconut oil to it. If you want to add it to your diet, it is recommended to try it out of a week and then try a week without it and compare the differences in your weight loss. If you are not satisfied with your weight loss, you can also try adjusting the ingredients and seeing if there are any improvements.

"Can I have Kombucha tea?"

For most people, it is fine to have kombucha tea in your diet. However, be careful of how much sugar is in the tea. Make sure the tea you have has no more than 2 grams of sugar. Kombucha tea has the potential to bump you out of ketosis, so experiment with it and see how it affects your body.

"Can I have fruit on a keto diet?"

Although fruits are considered healthy, they are actually very high in carbs and sugar, unlike the non-starchy vegetables. Therefore, in the keto diet, most fruits should be avoided. Certain berries are an exception; however, that can be consumed in small amounts. The ideal choices are blackberries, raspberries, and strawberries, which provide only 5-6 grams of carbs per 100 grams (or 3 ½ ounces). Most other fruits (including blueberries) contain double or triple this amount of carbs. It is also important to note that berries do not provide nutrients that cannot be found in other food options with fewer carbs, such as vegetables. This makes berries optional in the keto diet. If you have high insulin resistant, it might actually be better for you to avoid them anyway.

"How can I get rid of keto breath?"

As mentioned earlier, keto breath is a fruity smell similar to nail polish. This is the smell of acetone, which is a ketone body. It signifies that your body is burning lots of fat and is even converting fat to ketones to fuel your brain. Not everyone on a diet experiences this, with most people who do having it go away in a week or two. For the few individuals where it does not go away, here are a few suggestions:

- **Drink lots of fluids and get enough salt.** Keeping well hydrated has yet another benefit. If your mouth starts to feel dry, which often happens as you enter ketosis, it is due to your body making less saliva. This prevents bacteria from being washed away and can result in bad breath. Drinking enough water can help in this scenario.
- **Maintain good oral hygiene.** While brushing your teeth will not stop the fruity keto smell (as it comes from your lungs, not your mouth), it will at least prevent it from mixing with other smells.
- **Use a breath freshener regularly.** This can help mask the keto smell.
- **Reduce the degree of ketosis.** This is the easiest way to get rid of the smell if it becomes a long-term problem. This involves simply adding more carbs to your diet, 50-70 more grams per day can bring you out of ketosis. While this may limit the results produced by the low-carb diet, it may still be enough of a carb restriction to be effective.

"Can I eat a keto diet as a vegetarian or vegan?"

This type of diet can work for many types for non-meat eaters, but it depends on what other types of food are included in their diet. For instance, a lacto-ovo vegetarian eats dairy and eggs, whereas a lacto-vegetarian eats dairy but not eggs. A subset of vegetarians known as pescatarians have fish in their diet but cut out poultry and other meat. It is, therefore, doable to follow the keto diet, but it will be challenging to figure out the ideal meal plan. However, in terms of using a keto vegan diet, it is not a well-balanced or sustainable option. Vegans rely on a combination of grains, legumes, and seeds to get their essential vitamins and nutrients. This makes it very challenging on the keto diet.

"Is a keto diet safe for the kidneys?"

Yes! This is a common concern, due to the belief that a diet high in protein could be harmful to your kidneys. However, this fear is based on two misunderstandings:

- The keto diet is high in fat, **not** protein

- People with normal kidney function can handle excessive protein

The keto diet may actually be protective of your kidneys, especially if you have diabetes (due to lowering your amount of carbs in your diet and having better control of your blood sugars) [63, 64].

Chapter 10: Know Your Macros

Understanding your macros during this diet can cause a lot of confusion when you are trying to reach success. This chapter, with explanations from Dr. Eric Berge [65], will try to help clear up some of the more difficult concepts.

Macros refer to the percentage of carbohydrates, fats, and proteins you consume daily. These were mentioned in a previous chapter. If you were also to look up 'keto macros' in a Google search, the percentages you would most typically see **over 3 meals per day** are:

- 5% carbs
- 20% protein
- 75% fat [66]

These make up your 3 meals per day on the keto diet. However, when you throw in the feeding restriction from intermittent fasting, this changes the number of meals you have per day (down to 1-2) and overall percentages.

Side Note: *There is also another variable that should be included in your diet: the "non-starchy vegetables". These include your leafy-greens, broccoli, kale, etc., which would NOT be part of your carbohydrate section. This variable should make up about 5% of your diet, reducing the others accordingly.*

Let Us Use An Example

Say, over **3 meals a day,** you consume **1800 calories**. If you reduce down to **2 meals a day**, you should decrease to **1500 calories**, and if you are down to **1 meal a day,** it should be around **1200 calories**. The number of calories should be reduced at a specific **RATE**, due to your body retaining more nutrients from the fewer meals you have. This occurs because your body goes through metabolic adaptations the less frequently you eat. This will influence your macro percentages as well.

The rate itself does not have a variable related to the actual number of meals you have per day. The variable is determined by your unique body composition, age, sex, height, etc. It is unique to you!

So, let us break down the amounts of each variable, starting with the non-starchy vegetables. If you have **10 cups of salad per day**, **over 3 meals,** that would **be 3 1/3 cups**. However, if you are only having **2 meals per day**, due to the increased efficiency of your body, you will only need roughly **8 cups per day** or **4 cups per meal**. Then once you get down to **1 meal per day,** it will be reduced to **7 cups in that 1 meal**, on average.

In terms of the other carbohydrates (berries, tomatoes, beets, etc.), you want to aim to keep it between **20-50 grams per day** (ideally **below 30**

grams). You can keep this amount consistent, no matter the number of meals you are having per day. However, this **WILL** change your macro percentages, so it is important to keep that in mind.

Conversely, when looking at your total protein intake, the total **percentage** (20%) will stay the same no matter the number of meals you have per day. Therefore, unlike with carbohydrates, the **amount** you eat differs per number of meals. For example, on average, you would aim to have **4 oz of protein per meal** if you are having **3 meals a day**. This would change to **5oz per meal** if you are having **2 meals a day**, and **8oz per meal** if you are having **1 meal a day**.

Determining your amount of required fat intake can be more difficult than the other variables. At the beginning of your diet, your fat intake will be much higher and will slowly taper down as your progress, and your body adjusts to metabolizing your own fat storage. On average, you will want to consume roughly **140 grams of fat** if you are having **3 meals a day**, **113 grams** if you are having **2 meals a day**, and **86 grams** if you are having **1 meal a day** [65].

If you are still confused after this explanation, do not worry! These concepts are not the easiest to understand. Luckily, there are online resources that can help you calculate the amounts of each macro you should be consuming based on your demographic information, how active you are, and your ideal weight loss. One such resource is the **"Keto Calculator"**, which can be found at https://www.ruled.me/keto-calculator/. It provides a simple breakdown of your ideal daily intake of calories, fats, carbs, and proteins.

Chapter 11: Understanding Your Protein

In the last chapter, we looked at the overall amounts of macros you should be consuming during the keto diet to gain the most success. This chapter will now focus more specifically on **PROTEIN**.

First, a quick re-cap on body metabolism. As mentioned in previous chapters, the body will **FIRST** look for glucose, either from your diet or stored as glycogen, to metabolize for its energy source. This is the reason the keto diet limits your intake of carbs. Once your supply of glucose depletes, your body will then shift to metabolizing protein first before shifting to fats, which is the ultimate goal to bring your body to a state of ketosis. When your body is metabolizing protein, it will use your muscle protein **UNLESS** you consume enough protein in your diet. This is the reason it is important to consume a moderate amount of protein in this diet as well, not only high amounts of fat.

The amount of protein you need daily depends roughly on how much you weigh. Typically, you want to eat between **3 to 6 oz of protein per meal** or **0.36 to 0.7 grams per pound of body weight**. So, for example, if you weigh **185 lbs.**, you would want to eat **between 65 to 126 grams per day**. Then, if you are eating **3 meals a day,** you would have between **21 to 42 grams per meal**. These numbers will, of course, change if you are eating only 1 to 2 meals with intermittent fasting, due to the changes in your metabolism and your body adjusting to protect your muscle protein from being broken down. When you are consuming the correct amount of protein to prevent this breakdown, your body will then shift to metabolizing fat, becoming more efficient as time progresses.

Side note: you would not want to eat more protein than within this range, as this could lead to other problems. For instance, it could cause problems with your liver and kidneys, creating a strain on either and even causing kidney stones. Also, the excess protein will get converted to glucose and add fat to your body.

Remember, when you are buying food items and looking at weight in grams, make sure you are looking at the amount of **PROTEIN** in grams and not the **TOTAL** grams of the food item. For example, if you are buying some beef, which is listed as 113 grams and 4 oz, the amount of protein in it will be much less, probably closer to 26 grams. The largest portion of the total grams will be made up of water! It is also important to realize that your food items (fish, chicken, beef, etc.) will all have differing amounts of protein per unit of volume [67].

Chapter 12: Speeding Things Up

You may be wondering at this point: Is there any way you can speed up the process of weight loss? Getting your body to the necessary state of ketosis seems like a very long process! There are certainly some tricks, as described by Dr. Eric Berg [68, 69], which can help move things along at a faster pace to help you see results sooner.

Let Us Start With Speeding Up Intermittent Fasting

Potassium

This mineral is closely linked to your insulin levels. Our daily requirement for potassium is 4700 mg, and getting the correct amount helps prevent your body from secreting high amounts of insulin. This will, in turn, have a positive effect on your weight loss efforts, and other health issues involving memory, the cardiovascular system, and diabetes. Getting the right amount of potassium can be done by consuming large salads or enhancing your diet with the mineral.

Overeating

Because you are fasting, you might think you have to gorge yourself during your feeding period to get your calories and prevent hunger during your fasting period. A trick is to have a large salad sometime in between your two meals. This way, you are getting your greens, allowing yourself time to digest it, and not spiking your insulin in the process. This prevents you from feeling "stuffed" as well.

Do It Gradually

Do not feel you need to jump to a large fasting period too quickly! Let your body adapt over time, especially if you have a blood sugar issue such as hypoglycemia that would cause you to crash. A good recommendation is to start with 3 meals a day, without the snacks until you are comfortable. Then you can move to 2 meals a day, and slowly decrease your feeding window until it is where you want it to be.

Extra Sleep

Being stressed and tired makes you hungrier! This increases the hormone cortisol, which in turn increases your insulin levels and knocks you out of ketosis. A good way to avoid this is to ensure you get 7 to 8 hours of sleep **EACH DAY**. Throw in a nap during the day if you need to. Going for long walks will also help to keep your stress levels down, preventing the rise in your stress hormones and also helping you sleep.

Try High-Intensity Interval Training (HIIT)

This type of exercise is a full-body, high intensity, and high pulse-rate activity over a short duration. It is shown to have a highly positive effect on weight loss when combined with intermittent fasting. It is important when doing this activity to make sure you include lots of rest between the intervals, ideally doing it twice to three times a week to ensure adequate recovery. In terms of timing, you would want to do these intervals during your feeding period, either just before or just after your last meal, to ensure you do not drop your blood sugars too low [67].

Do Not Eat Until You Are Hungry

Even if you have entered your feeding period, if you are not hungry, do not force yourself to eat! Let your body tell you when to eat, not the other way around. If you are not hungry, your body is successfully sustaining itself on your own body fat for energy, so let that process continue until it needs a dietary source of energy. It is okay to eat at different times, so if you need to push your feeding period later in the day to when you are actually starting to feel hungry, that is perfectly acceptable!

Now How About Enhancing The Keto Diet
Reduce Your Carbs

As mentioned previously, your keto diet will typically include 20-50 grams of carbohydrates per day. One recommendation to greatly speed up your results is to **COMPLETELY** eliminate carbohydrates from your diet. While this is certainly extreme, it will bring your body to a state of ketosis that much quicker.

Avoid Low-Fat Protein

Ideally, you are going to want to consume food that combines your fat and protein naturally. If you are eating low-fat protein, you will then have to consume more food to get your required fat amount. Also, the leaner the protein, the higher the insulin spike.

Some lean forms of protein to **AVOID** include:

- Chicken
- Dairy
- Turkey
- Lean steak
- Lean fish
- Peanuts

Instead, you should be **FOCUSING ON** the fatty protein meals, including:

- Salmon
- Sardines
- Pork
- Hamburger
- Eggs

Be Careful About Adding Extra Fat

There are some forms of fat that you **SHOULD NOT** be adding to your diet, including **keto bombs** or **extra butter**. The types of fats that you **SHOULD** add include **avocado, olives, pecans**, or **almonds**. These fats include lots of nutrients as well and are considered healthier forms of fats.

Your body has a sort of "sweet spot" in terms of how much fat you should consume, and on average, it is around 75 grams. If you consume less than this amount (but no less than 50 grams), your body will start to metabolize its own body fat.

An example of a fat diet:

- 4 strips of bacon (13 grams)
- 2 eggs (10 grams)
- 4 oz steak (24 grams)
- 1 oz pecans (20 grams)

This would bring you to 67 grams of fat, which would encourage your body to metabolize its own fat.

Make Sure You Are Getting Your Leafy Greens

This topic has come up multiple times throughout this book, and it is because it is so important! They contain many of your required nutrients, including potassium, magnesium, and other vitamins. You also benefit from the **FIBER** from these vegetables. This fiber feeds the microbes throughout your digestive system, turning it into a very healthy fat called butyric acid. One benefit of this acid is its ability to help with insulin resistance, and potentially even lowering insulin levels.

Some Extra Tips:

- Consume about a teaspoon of sea salt on your meals daily
- Consume some electrolyte drinks, preferably those with high levels of potassium
- If you are having trouble consuming your salads, try adding apple cider vinegar, a little bit of sea salt, or balsamic vinaigrette to add some flavor. Make sure to get the kinds that are more bitter, however, and less sweet [69].

Chapter 13: The Dangers Of Deficiency

By this point, you should be getting comfortable with the ins and outs of the keto diet and intermittent fasting. **When** you eat and **what** you eat determine your overall success! There are, of course, certain things to keep in mind as you continue forward to ensure you stay healthy and happy.

The big thing to keep in mind, which has been mentioned in previous chapters, is **Nutrient Deficiency**. Ensuring what you eat is nutrient-dense is vital to keeping you strong and lively.

What Symptoms Should You Be Watching For?

Iron Deficiency

Iron is a vital component for the function of hemoglobin, a protein needed by red blood cells to transport oxygen. A lack of iron can lead to anemia due to a decrease in your red blood cell count. This is a blood disorder that causes *fatigue* and *weakness*, making it hard to function in your day-to-day activities.

Iron can be found in:

- Dark leafy greens (such as spinach, kale, swiss chard, and collard)
- Red meat (such as ground beef)
- Organ meat (such as liver)
- Egg yolks
- Shellfish (such as clams, mussels, and oysters)
- Beans (such as cooked kidney beans)
- Seeds (such as pumpkin, sesame, and squash)

Copper Deficiency

Copper is important for the development of red blood cells, as well as maintaining the nerve cells and the immune system. It also assists in the formation of collagen, absorption of iron, and production of energy. A lack of copper can cause symptoms such as *fatigue*, *frequent sickness, difficulty walking,* and *sensitivity to cold.*

Good sources of this mineral can be found in:

- Shellfish (such as oysters and lobster)
- Whole grains
- Beans (such as garbanzo)
- Nuts (such as cashews, hazelnuts, brazil, walnuts, pecans, and pine)
- Potatoes
- Dark leafy greens (such as turnip greens, spinach, and swiss chard)
- Dried fruits (such as figs, pears, peaches, apricots, mango, and dates)
- Cocoa
- Black pepper
- Yeast
- Organ meat (such as liver)

Vitamin A Deficiency

This vitamin is important for eye health and functioning, as well as reproductive health and the immune system. A deficiency can lead to *blindness in children* and an *increased mortality rate in pregnant women.*

It can be obtained from:
- Milk
- Eggs
- Green vegetables (such as kale and spinach)
- Orange vegetables (such as carrots and sweet potatoes)
- Reddish-yellow fruits (such as peaches and tomatoes)

Vitamin B1 (Thiamine) Deficiency

This vitamin is important for your nervous system, as well as your metabolism by helping convert carbs into energy. A lack of B1 causes *weight loss*, *fatigue*, *confusion*, and *short-term memory loss.*

You can avoid this deficiency by consuming:

- Eggs
- Legumes (such as green peas)
- Nuts (such as almonds, cashews, and walnuts)
- Seeds (such as sunflower seeds)
- Wheat germ
- Pork
- Cereals and grains fortified with thiamine
- Beans (such as navy, black, pinto, and lima)

Vitamin B3 (Niacin) Deficiency

This vitamin also aids in converting food to energy. A severe deficiency in B3 is called "pellagra", with symptoms including *diarrhea, dementia,* and *skin disorders.*

This vitamin is found in:

- Most animal proteins
- Peanuts

Vitamin B6 (Pyridoxine) Deficiency

This vitamin is crucial for brain development in babies and infants, as well as helping to bolster the immune system. A deficiency can result in *convulsions, hyperirritability,* and *peripheral neuropathy.*

This vitamin is found in:

- Chicken
- Fish (such as tuna)
- Potatoes
- Chickpeas
- Bananas

Vitamin B9 (Folate) Deficiency

This vitamin is involved with the creation of red blood cells and DNA, as well as brain development and the nervous system. It is **VITAL** for fetal development, as a lack of folate can result in *severe birth defects* involving the baby's brain and spinal cord.

You can find folate in:

- Beans and lentils
- Citrus fruits (such as oranges, grapefruit, lemons, and limes)
- Leafy greens (such as spinach, kale, and arugula)
- Asparagus
- Meat (including poultry and pork)
- Shellfish (such as oysters)
- Fortified grain products
- Whole grains

Vitamin B12 (Cobalamin) Deficiency

This is another vitamin involved in the formation of red blood cells. The observable symptoms of deficiency include *fatigue* and *weakness in extremities, dizziness, shortness of breath, weight loss, nausea* or *poor appetite, sore, red,* or *swollen tongue,* and *pale* or *yellowish skin*. **LONG-TERM** deficiency can lead to *difficulty walking, muscle weakness, irritability, dementia, depression,* and *memory loss.*

You can avoid these complications by consuming:

- Red meat and animal products
- Fortified plant-based milk
- Nutritional yeast
- Eggs
- Shellfish (such as clams and oysters)
- Organ meat (such as liver)

Vitamin C Deficiency

This vitamin is an important component of wound healing, as well as the facilitation of iron absorption. Signs of deficiency include *dry skin, slow-healing wounds, bleeding gums,* and *fatigue*. A poor diet, smoking, and drinking too much alcohol can lead to a decreased level of this vitamin.

The best sources are:

- Red and green peppers
- Oranges

- Strawberries
- Broccoli
- Kiwi
- Lemon
- Grapefruit
- Clams

Vitamin D Deficiency

This vitamin is essential for healthy bones and teeth and maintaining the correct amounts of calcium. An insufficient amount can lead to *osteoporosis*, causing fragile bones that break easily.

While your body can generate its own source of vitamin D from **sunlight**, it can also be found in:

- Fish liver oils (such as cod)
- Fatty fish
- Mushrooms
- Egg yolks
- Organ meat (such as liver)

Vitamin E Deficiency

This vitamin acts as an antioxidant and protects the body's cells from damage caused by free radicals. We can encounter these free radicals from the food we digest, as well as cigarette smoke, air pollution, and UV rays. It can also strengthen our immune system and prevent the development of blood clots. A deficiency can lead to *muscle weakness* and *hemolytic anemia* (the breakdown of our red blood cells).

It can be found naturally in:
- Sunflower seeds
- Almonds
- Green vegetables (such as spinach and broccoli)

Calcium Deficiency

This is another vitamin directly involved with strong bones and teeth development. As it is related to vitamin D levels, a lack of calcium can lead to *bone loss* and *osteoporosis*, although there is still some debate surrounding this. A deficiency can also lead to life-threatening *convulsions* and *abnormal heart rhythms*.

The best sources of calcium are found in:

- Dairy products (such as milk, yogurt, and cheese)
- Calcium-set tofu
- Small fish with bones (such as sardines)
- Dark green vegetables (such as kale, spinach, bok choy, and broccoli)

Potassium Deficiency

As mentioned previously, potassium is an important mineral for regulating insulin levels. It is also important for the proper function of muscles, maintaining fluid levels, health blood pressures, and regulating heartbeats. Symptoms of deficiency include *fatigue, muscle cramps, numbness, heart palpitations*, and *breathing difficulties*.

Sources of potassium include:

- Bananas
- Mushrooms
- Potatoes
- Green vegetables (such as peas, cooked broccoli, and spinach)
- Pumpkin

Iodine Deficiency

This nutrient is important for the production of thyroid hormones, which are essential for many bodily functions such as regulating calorie burn, heartbeat, body temperature, cell turnover, and brain health. A lack of iodine can lead to *fatigue, unexpected weight gain, dry skin,* and *hair loss.*

Common sources of this nutrient are:

- Dairy products (such as milk and cheese)
- Eggs
- Iodized salt

- Soymilk
- Fish (such as baked cod)
- Seaweed [70, 71, 72]

Chapter 14: Using Supplements

Obtaining your nutrients through your food is the healthiest option, as you are consuming them in their natural state. However, the keto diet cuts out many food options, which will limit where you can find all your required vitamins and minerals. Therefore, it would be a good idea to take supplements for the nutrients you may be missing. People have even found that some supplements can also reduce the adverse effects of the keto flu.

Which Supplements Would Be Beneficial?

Magnesium

This mineral helps to boost energy, regulate blood sugar levels, and support the immune system. You run the risk of not meeting your daily magnesium needs when on the keto diet, as must foods containing high magnesium, including **beans** and **fruits**, are also high in carbs. Supplementing **200-400 mg of magnesium** each day can help you meet your daily requirements, as well as *reducing symptoms* in the early stages of the keto diet, such as *muscle cramps, difficulty sleeping,* and *irritability* [73].

MCT Oil

These are medium-chain triglycerides, which are an immediate fuel source for your brain and muscles. The supplementation of the oil concentrates the MCT and increases your fate intake, helping you to stay in ketosis. Starting with **5 ml of MCT oil** will allow your body to adapt, before increasing to the suggested dose recommended on the supplement bottle [74].

Omega-3 Fatty Acids

These supplements contain eicosapentaenoic acid (EPA) and docosahexaenoic acid (DHA), which have been found to reduce inflammation and decrease the risk of heart disease and mental decline. If you wish to take an omega-3 supplement, it is recommended to choose a brand containing **500 mg of EPA and 1000 mg of DHA** per serving [75].

Vitamin D

As mentioned previously, it is important to meet your daily requirements of vitamin D to avoid unwanted side effects, including *osteoporosis*. Being on the keto diet does not directly increase your risk of vitamin D deficiency, but since the risk in common in all populations, taking a supplement is a good idea. To prevent osteoporosis, a daily of **400-1000 IU of vitamin D** is recommended [76].

Exogenous Ketones

These are commonly taken to increase your blood ketone levels, bringing you to a state of ketosis much quicker than when only using your endogenous source of ketones. The best exogenous ketone source contains **high-quality beta-hydroxybutyrate (BHB)**, as well as no fillers or additives [77].

Greens Powder

Adding this supplemental powder to your shakes and smoothies is an easy way to increase your vegetable intake, thus increasing your nutrient intake. Adequate greens intake fights inflammation, lowers disease risk, and helps overall bodily functions. Most powders contain a plant mixture of **spinach**, **spirulina**, **chlorella**, **kale**, **broccoli**, **wheatgrass**, and more [78].

Fiber

As mentioned previously, fiber is an important part of the digestive process. It is the indigestible part of the plants you eat, which helps keep your digestive system healthy and keeps you from becoming constipated. It is recommended that people should get **25-31 grams per day**. Although many food sources can supply fiber to your diet (i.e., nuts, seeds, avocado, and leafy greens) if you were to focus more so on consuming meat, seafood, eggs, and dairy, you may be missing out on your daily fiber requirements. Taking a fiber supplement can be beneficial, but it should be taken with plenty of water to avoid making constipation worse.

Digestive Enzymes

Enzymes are an important part of digestion as they help breakdown different parts of your food. Individuals who switch to the keto diet after previously eating a large number of carbs may experience trouble due to insufficient enzymes to assist in the digestion of their new diet. Symptoms can include *bloating*, *nausea*, *fatigue*, and *constipation* from the increased amount of fat consumption. Supplementing digestive enzymes, specifically **lipase** that specializes in digesting fat can help alleviate these symptoms. Adding **protease** and peptidase are good choices too, as they assist in protein breakdown.

L-theanine

This is an amino acid that is difficult to obtain from foods. The only food source is found in black or green tea, with varying amounts available depending on the type of tea and how it is brewed. Supplementing this amino acid has been shown to **improve sleep quality**, **decrease anxiety**, and **improve mental cognition**. While there is no recommended dosage, many products suggest **100-400 mg daily** [79].

Chapter 15: Getting Active

You have probably heard, "the key to weight loss is a change in diet as well as exercising." That being said, how do sports and exercise fit in with the keto diet and intermittent fasting? Are they safe to combine? What is the ideal timing for exercise during the day? In this chapter, we will address exercise in the context of **intermittent fasting** and then the **keto diet**.

Some Questions You May Have Surrounding Exercise With Intermittent Fasting

"Is it safe?"

In short, yes, it is safe to exercise while on this diet! It still helps decrease your risk of heart disease, obesity, and other physical and mental health conditions. You just need to be careful in your types of exercise to ensure they coincide well with your low-carb diet. Your performance during certain exercises may vary, and your intensity level may be lower than you are used to.

Four forms that most healthcare professionals recommend are:

- **Aerobic exercises** (such as **cycling**, **jogging**, or **swimming**) are lower intensity cardio that lasts over three minutes
- **Anaerobic exercises** (such as weightlifting or high-intensity interval training), which require short bursts of energy
- **Flexibility exercises** (such as **yoga** and simple **after-workout stretches**) help stretch out your muscles, support joints, and improve muscle range of motion. Increasing flexibility helps to prevent injuries
- **Stability exercises** (such as **balance** and **core training**) helps to improve your alignment, strengthen muscles, and control movement

It is important while exercising to **make sure you eat enough** to ensure you have enough nutrition to endure a workout. You will want to avoid forms of exercise that require more than **short bursts** of energy, as you will not be able to sustain them on this diet. Also, make sure to always **listen to your body**, and do not push yourself too far! Stay within the boundaries of what you can handle, and you will not cause yourself any harm [80, 81].

"When should you exercise?"

Intermittent fasting is going to be the component that will impact when you should schedule your workouts. Exercising in the **fasted stated** has shown to have its pros and cons. Some studies have suggested that exercising while fasting causes an increase in fat metabolism for fuel, as your stores of carbohydrates are already depleted. However, other studies have not observed a difference in fat loss when in a fasted vs. fed state [82, 83]. You also run the risk of losing muscle due to breakdown to use protein for fuel, and not performing as well due to decreased energy. That being said, this does not mean you cannot work out during the fasted state.

Here are two tips for doing it safely:

- **Stay hydrated and keep your electrolyte levels maintained.** This has been mentioned many times before, but it is important enough to mention again. Keeping yourself hydrated is especially important during your workout, where you will be losing even more water. You will also lose your electrolytes through your sweat, so hydrating with coconut water or electrolyte products helps replenish your needed water and electrolyte levels.
- **Eat a meal close to the workout.** You want to make sure your nutrition level is peaked after exercising to aid in recovery, such as building proteins and replenishing glycogen stores. In the fasted state, nutrients will be limited compared to consuming a meal before exercising [84].

"Is there a perfect time to exercise that maximize fat burning?"

The 'ideal time' for exercise to increase weight loss is considered to be in the **morning**. One of the reasons is linked to the previous point, being when you first wake up, your glucose levels are depleted, and your body will be forced to use fat stores of fuel. Research does not show that this results in a greater loss of body fat, though. However, actual benefits to exercising in the morning are seen due to your hormonal levels. **Testosterone**, which has been linked to fat loss and muscle gain, is observed to be higher in the morning and declines during the day. Other studies have shown that exercising in the morning can increase your hormones and neurotransmitters that are linked to increasing your energy levels, mood, and self-esteem. These all contribute to healthier decisions during the day! However, if exercising in the morning is impossible, either due to timing or fatigue, exercising in the afternoon or evening can be beneficial as well. **Ultimately, the perfect time is whenever you HAVE the time** [85]!

"Should you eat before or after your workout?"

As previously mentioned, the benefits of exercising while fasted are limited due to the mixed study results relating to overall fat loss. Furthermore, while fasting during short-duration exercise may not hamper performance, it has been observed that eating before long-duration exercise is beneficial. This is likely due to the increased available fuel source and nutrients, allowing the body to generate energy more easily. Therefore, the **type of exercise** will play a substantial role in when you do a workout relative to your feeding schedule [86].

"Does exercise affect my hunger level?"

It has been shown that, yes, exercise can suppress your appetite. Many studies have shown that regular workouts, specifically long sessions of aerobic exercise, can **suppress ghrelin**, a hormone that stimulates hunger. **Peptide YY**, a neurotransmitter that signals satiety, is also found to be **increased** for up to two to three hours after exercise. While these effects are temporary, they exemplify how exercise can help assist you in gaining success with the keto diet/

intermittent fasting. It has been shown that being only on a diet can increase levels of ghrelin and lower levels of peptide YY, which results in constant hunger. These are the complete opposite effects produced through exercising. **Exercising can help control your hunger, which will help you stick to the diet and gain successful weight loss. It can be a great help in bringing you to a state of ketosis, as it helps to deplete your stored glycogen, which your body will burn first for energy** [87].

Let Us Look At A Few Facts About Exercising While On The Keto Diet

High-Intensity workouts will be tougher on the keto diet.

These forms of exercise, which require short bursts of energy, are powered by your dietary carbohydrates. When it is stored as glycogen in your muscle cells, it can easily be tapped into as an energy source during intense movements, such as strength training, sprinting, etc. On the keto diet, your primary source of energy is obtained from burning fat, which is not metabolized as quickly as carbohydrates. This makes it less optimal as a fuel source for intense exercise, which requires energy very quickly. This results in limited performance on the keto diet. Lower-intensity workouts, such as cardio, are less affected.

You may feel less energized when starting the keto diet.

As your body switches from using carbohydrates to fats for its fuel source, those beginning the keto diet may initially feel less energized when working out. This is due to your body adapting to using this other form of energy. However, later on, your energy levels should increase and even surpass our normal levels as your body starts to metabolize your fats, especially when exercising [88].

You may start to burn calories quicker on the keto diet.

It has been shown that when the body replaces its fuel

source from carbs to fats, you will burn through calories quicker. A study in 2018 found that switching to a low-carbohydrate diet causes the body to burn approximately 250 more calories per day than if you had a high-carbohydrate, low-fat diet. This is primarily due to fat being more calorie-dense than carbohydrates [89].

Each gram of fat has nine calories, while a gram of protein or carbohydrate has four calories.

The keto diet helps you maintain muscle mass.

Being on the keto diet will help you to maintain your muscle mass, but not necessarily help you grow due to the lower number of calories and protein you take in each day. Also, the lesser amount of consumed carbohydrates will slow down the process. However, by at least maintaining your muscle mass, you will be burning a fair number of calories, even when you are not working out [88].

So, What Are Some Tricks To Maximize Your Results When You Are In Ketosis?

Plan your meals.

When you are exercising, you tend to eat more food due to your body using energy up at a faster rate. However, as mentioned earlier, energy breakdown is slower in a low-carbohydrate diet as opposed to a high one. This is why planning meals ahead is important, as having food prepared and available will help to avoid cravings and diet mishaps.

Keep watch of the number of carbs in your diet.

Expanding on the first point, it is normal for your body to crave carbohydrates when exercising due to them being quickly metabolized for energy. To maintain ketosis, however, you need to keep your dietary carbohydrates at the recommended minimum. Counting your calories will help you to keep you within your daily limit.

Have a balanced diet.

This was discussed in earlier chapters, describing how important it is to ensure you are still getting all your macronutrients to function optimally. This is done by eating nutrient-dense food (such as **leafy vegetables**, **nuts**, and **seeds**), which include the correct amount of fat, protein, and vitamins.

Find an exercise routine that works for you.

By having a full exercise routine, you will be able to target different parts of the body to make sure you are efficiently using your work out time. You do not even have to sign up at your local gym to exercise regularly – home workout routines are just as effective. If you are stuck, you can always get in touch with a fitness expert to help you find a routine that works best for you, or if you have any special fitness requirements.

Drink plenty of water.

This point comes up again and again throughout these chapters, which should hopefully tell you just how important it is! Proper hydration is especially important when exercising because your muscles require more water when undergoing strenuous activities. **So, drink up!**

Rest up.

The extra stress caused by exercising can be taxing on your body, increasing the importance that you get enough sleep daily to prevent fatigue. Six hours is generally the minimum sleep requirement for adults, but when exercising on the keto diet, you should aim to sleep at least 8 hours to allow your body the opportunity to recover properly.

Stay healthy.

Whether you are exercising on the keto diet or not, it is imperative you maintain a healthy lifestyle to get the most out of all your effort. This includes avoiding the use of drugs and other substances. Substance abuse can negatively affect your body's systems, not to mention, endanger your overall health [90].

Chapter 16: Keeping An Eye On The Calories

Specifically, with intermittent fasting, the main reason you will successfully lose weight is due to eating **fewer calories**. This is achieved through a restriction in your fasting period, as you will be preventing yourself from consuming excess calories throughout most of the day. As mentioned in previous chapters, however, it is important to make sure you are not **overeating** during your feed periods. The goal is to restrict your calorie intake, and gorging on food in a short period of time is counterintuitive. Having a restricted feeding period on top of a specific diet from the keto diet may cause difficulty in making sure you are getting the correct number of calories. It may be helpful to **track your food and calorie intake**. Many online calorie trackers can help you reach your goal! Here are some of the top trackers used today and their features:

MyFitnessPal (the premium version is $49.99/year)

Pros:

- Tracks your weight and uses it to calculate a recommended daily calorie intake
- Contains food diary and exercise log
- Clearly shows you how many calories you have consumed each day
- Shows the number you burned by exercising
- Extensive nutrition database
- Option to download recipes
- Has a barcode scanner to automatically enter the nutrition information for some food items
- Can "quick add" calories if too busy to add details of a meal

Cons:

- Calorie count might not be entirely accurate, as most foods are uploaded by other users
- Serving size may be hard to edit in the database

Lose It! (the premium version is $39.99/year)

Pros:

- Personalized recommendation for calorie intake based on your weight, height, age, and goals
- Comprehensive food database and food diary
- Easy to add new foods
- Shows weight changes through a graph
- Can set reminders to log your meals

Cons:

- Difficult to log home-cooked meals and calculate the nutritional value
- Does not track micronutrients

FatSecret

Pros:

- FREE!
- Contains a food diary, nutrition database, recipes, exercise log, weight chart and journal
- Includes a barcode scanner to help track some food items

- Shows total calorie intake, broken down into carbs, protein, and fat
- Shows monthly summary view of total calories consumed
- Can present net carbs, which can be handy for the keto diet

Cons:

- The interface can be a bit confusing to navigate

Cron-o-meter (gold upgrade is $3/month)

Pros:

- Offers exact serving sizes and exercise database
- Can select a customized profile for higher calorie needs if pregnant or lactating
- Can select a specific diet, which changes the macronutrient recommendations
- Shows total calories consumed and breakdown of carbs, fat, and protein per day
- Tracks micronutrients, like vitamins and minerals

- Syncs data from other health devices and imports weight, body fat percentage, sleep data, and activities

Cons:

- Food diary does not divide into meals
- Home-cooked recipes can only be added on the website, not the app. However, it will be available on the app afterward
- Website is free, but the app costs $2.99

SparkPeople (the premium version is $4.99/month or a one-time payment of $29.99)

Pros:

- Can copy and paste an entry into multiple days of the food diary, if you have eaten the same thing more than once
- Each day displays total calories, carbs, fats, and protein. Have the option to display as a pie chart

- Has one of the largest online food and nutrition databases

Cons:

- The site can appear overwhelming as it contains a lot of information
- The content is spread across multiple apps (i.e., one app for pregnant women, one for recipes, etc.)
- Some difficulties logging foods into the app [91]

Chapter 17: An Example Routine

You have made it to the last chapter of the book! By this point, you have covered the ins and outs of the keto diet and intermittent fasting, and how to use them together successfully. You have got all the tools, now to finish up let us look at a **Typical Daily Routine**. *We will use the* **16:8 intermittent fasting model**, *for a participant with a* **9 am to 5 pm, 5 days a week work schedule**.

To start, you will need to determine what your ideal feeding period is. This will involve eliminating a meal, so you will need to decide whether you want to skip **breakfast** or **supper**? For an 8-hour feeding period, both options can potentially look like the following:

Skipping Breakfast

On average, supper time is usually between 6 pm and 7 pm. If we use the lower end (7 pm) as your last meal for the day, this means your first meal of the day would be at 11 am, 2 hours after arriving at work.

Skipping Supper

On average, a 9am work start means breakfast between 7 am and 8 am. Using the lower end (8 am) as your first meal means you can eat until 4 pm, an hour before you finish work.

Many people might feel they need the energy boost first thing in the morning to start their day, which means they would most prefer skipping supper instead of breakfast. For that reason, we will use the **skipping supper** *choice in this routine.*

When first starting this routine, it would be a good idea to start the intermittent fasting portion slowly. For the first day, start with a 12-hour feeding period. Therefore, if you start eating at **8 am**, have your last meal at **8 pm**. Then over the following days, slowly decrease your feeding window by an hour. Each day, you can also introduce healthy habits to help you succeed in this diet. For example:

Day 1 Feeding Period

- 8 am to 8 pm
- **Goal**: Picking your feeding period
- Make sure skipping your supper instead of your breakfast is the optimal choice for you and your success

Day 2 Feeding Period

- 8 am to 7 pm
- **Goal**: Start focusing on eating more whole foods
- Start eliminating sugars, processed food and empty carbs from your diet

Day 3 Feeding Period

- 8 am to 6 pm
- **Goal**: Create a reward system to keep up your motivation

- Your reward system should be something related to relaxing, socializing, food or playing, which are your primal needs

Day 4 Feeding Period

- 8 am to 5 pm
- **Goal**: Make sure you are getting a high protein breakfast
- You will have been fasting for 11 hours by this point, and breaking your fast with a high protein meal will support your weight loss goal

Day 5 Feeding Period

- 8 am to 4 pm
- **Goal**: Drink black coffee when hungry
- As previously mentioned, coffee can help suppress your appetite making it easier to get through your fasting period. However, make sure it is **BLACK** coffee without any additives such as creamers or sugar, which are empty carbs.

Day 6 (And Onwards) Feeding Period

- 8 am to 4 pm
- **Goal**: Go for a walk during your fast
- Not only does it improve your overall fitness, but it will help you take your mind off your hunger. It also helps with your overall weight loss

Once you reach Day 5-6, you should be within your ideal feeding period. Now you just need to maintain this schedule [92]*!*

Switching gears, now you need to start planning your keto diet meals for your fasting period. Some things to keep in mind that we have covered in earlier chapters include:

- Making sure you are getting your daily calories
- Eating nutrient-dense foods to prevent vitamin deficiency
- Drinking plenty of water

- Getting lots of rest

Here Is A List Of Healthy Keto-Friendly Meals To Break Your Fast With

- **Bacon and eggs**, with cherry tomatoes and fresh parsley
- **A frittata** made with bacon, eggs, fresh spinach, whipped cream, and shredded cheese
- **An omelet** made with eggs, shredded cheese, onions, and mushrooms
- **Boiled eggs** with mayonnaise and avocado
- **Mexican scrambled eggs**, with scallions, jalapeños, tomatoes, and shredded cheese
- **A western omelet**, with eggs, sour cream, shredded cheese, smoked deli ham, onions, and green bell peppers
- **Flourless egg and cottage cheese breakfast muffins**, with green onions, hemp seeds, parmesan cheese, almond meal, flaxseed meal, and yeast flakes

- **Cream cheese pancakes**, with eggs, stevia, and cinnamon
- **Crustless quiche**, with mushrooms, garlic, frozen spinach, eggs, milk, feta cheese, grated parmesan, and mozzarella
- **Coconut chia pudding**, with chia seeds, and honey
- **Low-carb waffles**, with eggs, coconut flour, milk, and stevia
- **Cowboy breakfast skillet**, with breakfast sausage, sweet potatoes, eggs, avocados, cilantro, hot sauce, and raw cheese
- **Bacon pancakes**, with coconut flour, gelatin, and chives
- **Avocado stuffed with smoked salmon and egg**, with chili flakes and fresh dill
- **Paleo sausage egg 'McMuffin'**, with ghee, pork breakfast sausage, and guacamole [93, 94]

A nutrient-filled meal is an ideal way to enter your feeding period, giving you the energy to start your day. Next, you will want to have some keto-friendly snacks available throughout the day between your meals. On top of **drinking plenty of water** or a **few cups of coffee**, here are a few options to keep you satisfied:

- Almonds and cheddar cheese
- Guacamole with low-carb veggies
- Trail mix made with unsweetened coconut, nuts, and seeds
- Coconut chips
- Kale chips
- Olives and sliced salami
- Celery and peppers with herbed cream cheese dip
- Berries with whipped cream
- Jerky
- Cheese roll-ups
- Parmesan crisps
- Macadamia nuts
- Leafy greens with high-fat dressing and avocado
- Smoothie made with coconut milk, cocoa and avocado [66]

And finally, your last meal of the day! It is just as

important as your first meal of the day, as it will need to keep you satisfied until you break your fast the following morning. Here are some examples of what you can make:

- **Loaded cauliflower**, with sour cream, grated cheddar cheese, bacon crumbles, snipped chives, and garlic powder
- **Zucchini pasta**, with chicken, pistachios, garlic, scallions, mint leaves, and lemon juice
- **Shrimp**, with cauliflower, grits, and arugula
- **Cheese shell taco cups**, with sour cream, and salsa made from diced tomatoes, red onions, jalapeños, and cilantro
- **Shrimp zoodles**, with zucchini, lemon, minced garlic, red pepper flakes, and fresh parsley
- **Blackened salmon with avocado salsa**, with diced red onions, diced jalapeños, chopped cilantro, chopped parsley, diced cucumber, and lemon
- **Greek yogurt chicken salad stuffed peppers**, with Dijon mustard, fresh parsley, sliced celery,

sliced scallions, cherry tomatoes, English cucumbers, and bell peppers
- **Keto pizza**, with eggs, parmesan cheese, psyllium husk powder, mozzarella cheese, tomato sauce, and chopped basil
- **Turkey and bacon wraps with basil mayo**, with lemon, garlic, lettuce, avocados, and tomatoes
- **Chicken and snap pea stir fry**, with sliced scallions, minced cloves, sliced bell peppers, sesame seeds, and fresh cilantro
- **Turkey meatball and kale soup**, with eggs, coconut or almond flour, crushed garlic, fresh herbs, onions, chopped carrots, bay leaves, and red pepper flakes
- **Thai chicken lettuce wraps**, with red curry paste, minced ginger, minced garlic, sliced red bell peppers, chopped green onions, shredded cabbage, hoisin sauce, and chopped basil
- **Gazpacho**, with diced tomatoes, diced cucumber, diced red bell pepper, garlic clove, minced red onion, chopped basil, chopped cherry tomatoes, and olive oil

- **Grilled spicy lime shrimp**, with olive oil, minced garlic, chili powder, ground cumin, and red pepper flakes
- **Cauliflower chowder**, with diced onion, garlic cloves, diced carrots, vegetable broth, dried oregano, cream cheese, olive oil, and cooked bacon [95]

Once you have had your supper, it is time to start the fast. This is where your pre-planned distractions come in handy! One of the best distractions that also helps with your weight loss efforts is **exercise**. Be it going for a walk, playing your favorite sport, or doing a low-intensity cardio work out at the gym, it is a great way to help you pass the time and keep your hunger at bay.

Conclusion

Congratulations on the completion of this book!

Intermittent fasting and the ketogenic diet have both been proven in the scientific literature as effective methods for stimulating weight loss, as well as lowering your cholesterol and overall health. Intermittent fasting helps you to determine **when** you will eat, whereas the keto diet helps you figure out **what** you will be eating and in what quantities when divided into protein, carbs, and fats. Combining the two methods allows a quicker entrance to a state of ketosis and, ultimately faster weight loss.

When you are awake and on your fast, it is important to remember to keep yourself occupied to help ignore any feelings of hunger. Sports, reading, movies, anything to keep your mind on other tasks! An occupied mind helps the time go quicker until you can eat again. Keeping yourself hydrated helps as well. Not only is it important for your health, but drinking water helps with hunger pangs. The occasional black coffee can help do the trick too. However, even the most dedicated dieter can fall off their schedule. The important thing is not to give up. An adjustment can get you right back on track, and a positive attitude can help you continue onwards successfully. Everyone makes mistakes, do not let it get you down! Making the adjustments for these two methods can present another challenge. Initially, you will most likely feel quite hungry during your fasting periods, and you may miss eating your carbohydrates as often as you did previously. The important thing is to stick with it. With regards to fasting, easing into it while slowly decreasing feeding periods over the first week will help the adjustment period be more manageable. Within a few days, your body will adapt. You can also replace your favorite carbs with other foods that mimic them, making this diet switch even easier.

It is important in the keto diet to ensure you are getting all your required nutrition. It is easy to develop different kinds of nutrient deficiencies if you are not careful. Knowing which food types supply your vitamins and minerals helps prevent these deficiencies and keeps your body healthy and functioning properly. On the opposite end, you also need to watch your total calorie intake to make sure it does not increase. Due to the intermittent fasting, you might feel that you need to gorge yourself during the feeding period to help you make it through the fasting period. The opposite is required, as decreasing your total number of consumed calories is what will help you succeed in weight loss. To complement these methods, incorporating exercise into the mix will help enhance your weight loss efforts even more. Exercises routines that require more than short bursts of energy may be too challenging with intermittent fasting and the keto diet, but introducing the right types of exercise will help keep you healthy and improve your fitness.

We thank you for letting us help you with your weight loss journey and feel confident that with the help of our tips and tricks, you will be well on your way to a happier,

healthier you!

References

1. Barnosky, A. R., Hoddy, K. K., Unterman, T. G., et al. "Intermittent fasting vs. daily calorie restriction for type 2 diabetes prevention: a review of human findings." Transl Res. 2014; 164(4): 302-11.
2. Cahill, G. F. "Fuel Metabolism in Starvation." Annu Rev Nutr. 2005; 26: 1-22.
3. Varady, K. A., Bhutani, S., Klempel, C. M., et al. "Alternate day fasting for weight loss in normal weight and overweight subjects: a randomized controlled trial." Nutr J. 2013; 12(1): 146.
4. Bhutani, S., Klempel, M. C., Kroeger, C. M., et al. "Alternate day fasting and endurance exercise combine to reduce body weight and favorably alter plasma lipids in obese humans." Obesity (Silver Spring). 2013; 21(7): 1370-9.
5. Heilbronn, L. K., Smith, S. R., Martin, C. K., et al. "Alternate-day fasting in nonobese subjects: effects on body weight, body composition, and energy metabolism." Am J Clin Nutr. 2005; 81(1): 69-73.
6. Lantz, H., Peltonen, M., Agren, L., et al. "Intermittent version on-demand use of a very low-

calorie diet: a randomized 2-year clinical trial." J Intern Med. 2003; 253(4): 463-71.

7. Harie, M. N., Pegington, M., Mattson, M. P., et al. "The effects of intermittent or continuous energy restriction on weight loss and metabolic disease risk markers: a randomized trial in young overweight women." International Journal of Obesity. 2011; 35(5): 714-27.

8. Collier, R. "Intermittent fasting: the science of going without." CMAJ. 2013; 185(9): E363-4.

9. Byrne, N. M., Sainsbury, A., King, N. A., et al. "Intermittent energy restriction improves weight loss efficiency in obese men: the MATADOR study." Int J Obes (Lond). 2018; 42(20: 129-38.

10. Harvie, M. N., Sims, A. H., Pegington, M., et al. "Intermittent energy restriction induces changes in breast gene expression and systemic metabolism." Breast Cancer Research. 2016; 18(1): 57.

11. Horne, B. D., Cox, J. E., Muhlestein, J. B., et al. "Abstract 13421: 24-Hour Water-Only Fasting Acutely Reduces Trimethylamine N-Oxide: the

FEELGOOD Trial." Circulation. 2014; 130(Suppl 2).

12. Stote, K. S., Baer, D. J., Spears, K., et al. "A controlled trial of reduced meal frequency without caloric restriction in healthy, normal-weight, middle-aged adults." Am J Clin Nutr. 2007; 85(4): 981-8.

13. Gunnars, K. (2017, June 4). "6 Popular Ways to Do Intermittent Fasting." Healthline. Retrieved from https://www.healthline.com/nutrition/6-ways-to-do-intermittent-fasting

14. Leonard, J. (2018, June 28). "Seven ways to do intermittent fasting." MedicalNewsToday. Retrieved from https://www.medicalnewstoday.com/articles/322293.php

15. Sogawa, H. and Kubo, C. "Influence of short-term repeated fasting on the longevity of female (NZB x NZW) F1 mice." Mech Ageing Dev. 2000; 115(1-2): 61-71.

16. Link, R. (2018, September 4). "16/8 Intermittent Fasting: A Beginner's Guide." Healthline. Retrieved

from https://www.healthline.com/nutrition/16-8-intermittent-fasting

17. Burton, M. J., Rolls, E. T., and Mora, F. "Effects of hunger on the responses of neurons in the lateral hypothalamus to the sight and taste of food." Experimental Neurology. 1976; 51(30): 668-77.

18. Poinier, A. C., Romito, K., Gabica, M. J., et al. (2018. June 25). "Hunger, Fullness, and Appetite Signals." Michigan Medicine: University of Medicine. Retrieved from https://www.uofmhealth.org/health-library/aa155258

19. Egecioglu, E., Skibicka, K. P., Hansson, C., et al. "Hedonic and incentive signals for body weight control." Metabolic Disorders. 2011; 12(3): 141-51.

20. Petrucci K. and Flynn, P. (2013, December). "Why water is so important when fasting." Fast Diets For Dummies. Retrieved from https://www.dummies.com/health/nutrition/weight-loss/why-water-is-so-important-when-fasting/

21. CBHS Health Fund. (2014, October 6). "The Importance of Staying Hydrated." Retrieved from

https://www.cbhs.com.au/health-well-being-blog/blog-article/2014/10/06/the-importance-of-staying-hydrated

22. Pollock, T. (2019, February 22). "Put Down That Water Bottle! 10 Creative Tricks To Stay Hydrated." MindBodyGreen. Retrieved from https://www.mindbodygreen.com/0-14453/put-down-that-water-bottle-10-creative-tricks-to-stay-hydrated.html

23. Laurence, E. (2018, November 14). "Is coffee, um, *allowed* while you're intermittent fasting?" Well+Good. Retrieved from https://www.wellandgood.com/good-food/intermittent-fasting-coffee/

24. Hirshkowitz, M., Whiton, K., Albert, S. M., et al. "National Sleep Foundation's sleep time duration recommendations: methodology and results summary." Sleep Health. 2015; 1(1): 40-3.

25. Antelmi, E., Vinai, P., Marcatelli, M., et al. "Nocturnal eating is part of the clinical spectrum of restless legs syndrome and an underestimated risk

factor for increased body mass index." Sleep Med. 2014; 15(2): 168-72.

26. Yamaguchi, M., Uemura, H., Katsuura-Kamano, S., et al. "Relationship of dietary factors and habits with sleep-wake regularity." Asia Pac J Clin Nutr. 2013; 22(3): 457-65.

27. Michalsen, A., Schlegel, F., Rodenbeck, A., et al. "Effects of short-term modified fasting on sleep patterns and daytime vigilance in non-obese subjects: results of a pilot study." Ann Nutr Metab. 2003; 47(5): 194-200.

28. Azrin, N. H., Kellen, M. J., Brooks, J., et al. "Relationship Between Rate of Eating and Degree of Satiation." Child Family Behavior Therapy. 2008; 30(4): 355-64.

29. Oshin, M. "11 Lessons Learned from 4 years of Intermittent Fasting: The Good and Bad." Healthy eating, Self Improvement, Strength Training. Retrieved from https://mayooshin.com/intermittent-fasting-lessons-learned/

30. Jarreau, P. B. (2018, March 21). "Time-Restricted Feeding: How and When You Break Your Fast Matters". Medium. Retrieved from https://medium.com/lifeomic/time-restricted-feeding-how-and-when-you-break-your-fast-matters-f241d40950f3

31. Petrucci, K. and Flynn, P. "9 Ways to Stave Off Hunger When fasting." Fast Diets for Dummies. Retrieved from https://www.dummies.com/health/nutrition/weight-loss/9-ways-to-stave-off-hunger-when-fasting/

32. Sakamoto, K. and Grunewald, K. K. "Beneficial Effects of Exercise on Growth of Rats During Intermittent Fasting." The Journal of Nutrition. 1987; 117(2): 390-5.

33. Volpe, A. (2019, April 18). "The Easier Way to Do Intermittent Fasting." Elemental. Retrieved from https://elemental.medium.com/the-easier-way-to-do-intermittent-fasting-9a9c60ba2e96

34. Swink, T. D., Vining, E. P., and Freeman, J. M. "The ketogenic diet: 1997." Advances in Pediatrics. 1997; 44: 297-329.

35. Badman, M. K., Kennedy, A. R., Adams, A. C., et al. "A very low-carbohydrate ketogenic diet improves glucose tolerance in ob/ob mice independently of weight loss." Am J Physiol Endocrinol Metab. 2009; 297(5): E1197-204.

36. Yancy, W. S. Jr., Olsen, M. K., Guyton, J. R., et al. "A low-carbohydrate, ketogenic diet versus a low-fat diet to treat obesity and hyperlipidemia: a randomized, controlled trial." Ann Intern Med. 2004; 140(10): 769-77.

37. Sondike, S. B., Copperman, N., and Jacobson, M. S. "Effects of a low-carbohydrate diet on weight loss and cardiovascular risk factor in overweight adolescents." The Journal of Pediatrics. 2003; 142(3): 221-2.

38. Dyson, P. A., Beatty, S., and Matthews, D. R. "A low-carbohydrate diet is more effective in reducing body weight than healthy eating in bother diabetic and non-diabetic subjects." Diabet Med. 2007; 24(12): 1430-5.

39. Foster, G. D., Wyatt, H. R., Hill, J. O., et al. "A randomized trial of a low-carbohydrate diet for obesity." N Engl J Med. 2003; 348(21): 2082-90.
40. Willi, S. M., Oexmann, M. J., Wright, N. M., et al. "The Effects of a High-protein, Low-fat, Ketogenic Diet, on Adolescents with Morbid Obesity: Body Composition, Blood Chemistries, and Sleep Abnormalities." Pediatrics. 1998; 101(1 Pt 1): 61-7.
41. Spritzler, F. (2017, January 23). "16 Foods to Eat on a Ketogenic Diet." Healthline. Retrieved from https://www.healthline.com/nutrition/ketogenic-diet-foods
42. Morris, M. C., Evans, D. A., Tangney, C. C., et al. "Fish consumption and cognitive decline with age in a large community study." Arch Neurol. 2005; 62(12): 1849-53.
43. Zhang, X., Shu, X. O., Xiang, Y. B., et al. "Cruciferous vegetable consumption is associated with a reduced risk of total and cardiovascular disease mortality." Am J Clin Nutr. 2011; 94(1): 240-6.

44. Whigham, L. D., Watras, A. C., and Schoeller, D. A. "Efficacy of conjugated linoleic acid for reducing fat mass: a meta-analysis in humans." Am J Clin Nutr. 2007; 85(5): 1203-11.

45. López Ledesma, R., Frati, Munari, A. C., Hernández, B. C., et al. "Monounsaturated fatty acid (avocado) rich diet for mild hypercholesterolemia." Arch Med Res. 1996; 27(4): 519-23.

46. Harber, M. P., Schenk, S., Barkan, A. L., et al. "Effects of dietary carbohydrate restriction with high protein intake on protein metabolism and the somatotropic axis." J Clin Endocrinol Metab. 2005; 90(9): 5175-81.

47. Ratliff, J., Leite, J. O., De Ogburn, R., et al. "Consuming eggs for breakfast influences plasma glucose and ghrelin, while reducing energy intake during the next 24 hours in adult men." Nutr Res. 2010; 30(2): 96-103.

48. Assunção, M. L., Ferreira, H. S., dos Santos, A. F., et al. "Effects of dietary coconut oil on the biochemical anthropometric profiles of women

presenting abdominal obesity." Lipids. 2009; 44(7): 593-601.

49. Tremblay, A., Doyon, C., and Sanchez, M. "Impact of yogurt on appetite control, energy balance, and body composition." Nutr Rev. 2015; 73(Suppl 1): 23-7.

50. Perdomo, L., Beneit, N., Otero, Y. F. "Protective role of oleic acid against cardiovascular insulin resistance and in the early and late cellular atherosclerotic process." Cardiovasc Diabetol. 2015; 14: 75.

51. Grosso, G. and Estruch, R. "Nut consumption and age-related disease." Maturitas. 2016; 84: 11-6.

52. Skorvankova, S., Sumczynski, D., Mlcek, J., et al. "Bioactive Compounds and Antioxidants Activity in Different Types of Berries." Int J Mol Sci. 2015; 16(10): 24673-706.

53. Warensjö, E., Smedman, A., Stegmayr, B., et al. "Stroke and plasma markers of milk fat intake—a prospective nested case-control study." Nutr J. 2009; 8: 21.

54. Yu, K., Ke, M. Y., Li, W. H., et al. "The impact of soluble dietary fiber on gastric emptying, postprandial blood glucose and insulin in patients with type 2 diabetes." Asia Pac J Clin Nutr. 2014; 23(2): 210-8.

55. Hagiwara, K., Goto, T., Araki, M., et al. "Olive polyphenol hydroxytyrosol prevents bone loss." Eur J Pharmacol. 2011; 662(1-3): 78-84.

56. van Dieren, S., Uiterwaal, C. S., vander Schouw, Y. T., et al. "Coffee and tea consumption and risk of type 2 diabetes." Diabetologia. 2009; 52(12): 2561-9.

57. Grassi, D., Desideri, G., Necozione, S., et al. "Blood pressure is reduced and insulin sensitivity increase in glucose-intolerant, hypertensive subjects after 15 days of consuming high-polyphenol dark chocolate." J Nutr. 2008; 138(9): 1671-6.

58. Lodge, S. (2018, August 19). "The Targeted Keto Diet vs. Other Keto Diets: How Does It Measure Up?" PerfectKeto. Retrieved from https://perfectketo.com/keto-diet-types/

59. Gustin, A. (2018, August 25). "Intermittent Fasting and Keto: Can You Do Them Both?" Perfect Keto. Retrieved from https://perfectketo.com/intermittent-fasting-and-keto/

60. Migala, J. (2019, January 29). "Intermittent Fasting on Keto: What to Know Before Combining the Diets for Weight Loss." Everyday Health. Retrieved from https://www.everydayhealth.com/ketogenic-diet/intermittent-fasting-keto-how-it-works-benefits-risks-more/

61. Berg, E. "Making it Super Easy to Stick to Your Keto and Intermittent Fasting Plan". YouTube. 12 February, 2018. https://www.youtube.com/watch?v=3IMIzZeyO8Y

62. Matthews, M. (2018, October 24). "26 Keto-Friendly Replacements for High-Carb Foods." Men's Health. Retrieved from https://www.menshealth.com/nutrition/a24166260/keto-diet-substitutes/

63. Berg, E. "Intermittent Fasting & Ketosis: 15 Common Questions & Answers." YouTube. 26 May, 2017. https://www.youtube.com/watch?v=DFsmgwiGyNI

64. Eenfeldt, A. and Spritzler, F. (2019, September 2). "What is a keto diet, and other common questions." DietDoctor. Retrieved from https://www.dietdoctor.com/low-carb/keto/common-questions#howdoyouknowhenyourbodyisinketosis

65. Berg, E. "The Ketogenic Diet: Calorie Confusions & Details When Doing Keto and Intermittent Fasting." YouTube. 8 February, 2018. https://www.youtube.com/watch?v=vB2EtclQLRA

66. Kubala, J. (2018, August 21). "A Keto Diet Meal Plan and Menu That Can Transform Your Body." Healthline. Retrieved from https://www.healthline.com/nutrition/keto-diet-meal-plan-and-menu

67. Berg, E. "How Many Grams of Protein on a Keto & Intermittent Fasting Plan?" YouTube. 10 March, 2018.
https://www.youtube.com/watch?v=bLGlP8T7zUo
68. Berg, E. "5 Tricks to Make Intermittent Fasting Work Faster." YouTube. 27 June, 2017.
https://www.youtube.com/watch?v=SYVvqY-evqQ
69. Berg, E. "Keto on Steroids / 5 Extreme Weight Loss Hacks." YouTube. 22 September, 2018.
https://www.youtube.com/watch?v=mlJRSebJoXA
70. Olsen, N. (2018, February 13). "Nutritional Deficiencies (Malnutrition)." Healthline. Retrieved from
https://www.healthline.com/health/malnutrition
71. Peters, St. (2019, August 20). "Nearly 10% of Americans have a nutritional deficiency. These are the most common." USA Today. Retrieved from https://www.usatoday.com/story/news/health/20

19/08/20/most-common-nutritional-deficiencies/39976101/

72. Bjarnadottir, A. (2019, May 21). "7 Nutrient Deficiencies That Are Incredibly Common". Healthline. Retrieved from https://www.healthline.com/nutrition/7-common-nutrient-deficiencies

73. Gröber, U., Schmidt, J., and Kisters, K. "Magnesium in Prevention and Therapy." Nutrients. 205; 7(9): 8199-226.

74. Liu, Y. M. and Wang, H. S. "Medium-chain triglyceride ketogenic diet, an effective treatment for drug-resistance epilepsy and a comparison with other ketogenic diets." Biomed J. 2013; 36(1): 9-15.

75. Nichols, P. D., McManus, A., Krail, K., et al. "Recent Advances in Omega-3: Health Benefits, Sources, Products and Bioavailability." Nutrients. 2014; 6(9): 3727-33.

76. WebMD. (2018). "Vitamin D." Retrieved from https://www.webmd.com/vitamins/ai/ingredient mono-929/vitamin-d

77. Gustin, A. (2018, August 21). "Using Supplements on Keto: The Top 16 and Why You Need Them." Perfect Keto. Retrieved from https://perfectketo.com/using-supplements-on-keto/

78. Kubala, J. (2018, June 28). "The 9 best Keto Supplements." Healthline. Retrieved from https://www.healthline.com/nutrition/best-keto-supplements

79. Berry, J. (2019, August 29). "The 7 best supplements for keto diets." MedicalNewsToday. Retrieved from https://www.medicalnewstoday.com/articles/326204.php

80. Dowell, M. (2018, September 4). "Can Your Exercise on the Keto Diet? Best Workouts for Weight Loss." CheatSheet Showbiz. Retrieved from https://www.cheatsheet.com/health-fitness/can-you-exercise-on-the-keto-diet-best-workouts-for-weight-loss.html/

81. Gustin, A. (2018, September 15). "How to Exercise When You're in Ketosis." PerfectKeto. Retrieved

from https://perfectketo.com/how-to-exercise-in-ketosis/

82. Bachman, J. L., Deitrick, R. W., and Hillman, A. R. "Exercising in the Fasted State Reduced 24-Hour Energy Intake in Active Male Adults." J Nutr Metab. 2016; 2016: 1984198.

83. Melanson, E. L., MacLean, P. S., and Hill, J. O. "Exercise improves fat metabolism in muscle but does not increase 24-h fat oxidation." Exerc Sport Sci Rev. 2009; 37(2): 93-101.

84. Stokes, T., Hector, A. J., and Morton, R. W. "Recent Perspectives Regarding the Role of Dietary Protein for the Promotion of Muscle Hypertrophy with Resistance Exercise Training." Nutrients. 2018; 10(20): E180.

85. Fetters, K. A. (2018, July 20). "Does It Matter What Time of Day You Exercise to Lose Weight?" Health. Retrieved from https://health.usnews.com/wellness/fitness/articles/2018-07-20/does-it-matter-what-time-of-day-you-exercise-to-lose-weight

86. Tinsley, G. (2018, May 27). "Should You Eat Before or After Working Out?" Healthline. Retrieved from https://www.healthline.com/nutrition/eating-before-or-after-workout
87. Stensel, D. "Exercise, appetite and appetite-regulating hormones: implications for food intake and weight control." Ann Nutr Metab. 2010; 57(Suppl 2): 36-42.
88. Dolan, M. (2019, June 17). "6 Things You Need to Know About Exercising on the Keto Diet." EveryDayHealth. Retrieved from https://www.everydayhealth.com/fitness/what-keto-diet-will-your-workout/
89. Ebbeling, C. B., Feldman, H. A., Klein, G. L., et al. "Effects of a low-carbohydrate diet on energy expenditure during weight loss maintenance: randomized trial." BMJ. 2018; 363.
90. Lucas, N. (2018, September 11). "7 Ways to Exercise Better When You Are In Ketosis." The Box. Retrieved from https://www.theboxmag.com/crossfit-training/7-ways-to-exercise-better-when-you-are-in-ketosis

91. Bjarnadottir, A. (2018, October 3). "The 5 Best Calorie Counter Websites and Apps." Healthline. Retrieved from https://www.healthline.com/nutrition/5-best-calorie-counters
92. Sinkus, T. (2019). "21 Day Intermittent Fasting Plan." 21 Day Hero. Retrieved from https://21dayhero.com/intermittent-fasting-daily-plan/
93. Eenfeldt, A. (2019, January 1). "Top low-carb and keto egg breakfasts". Diet Doctor. Retrieved from https://www.dietdoctor.com/low-carb/recipes/breakfasts/eggs
94. Gunnars, K. (2017, May 30). "18 Delicious Low-carb Breakfast Recipes." Healthline. Retrieved from https://www.healthline.com/nutrition/18-low-carb-breakfast-recipes
95. Champion, L. (2018, July 16). 40 Ketogenic Dinner Recipes You Can Make in 30 Minutes or Less. Pure Wow. Retrieved from https://www.purewow.com/food/ketogenic-dinner-recipes

Disclaimer

The information contained in this book and its components, is meant to serve as a comprehensive collection of strategies that the author of this book has done research about. Summaries, strategies, tips and tricks are only recommendations by the author, and reading this book will not guarantee that one's results will exactly mirror the author's results.

The author of this book has made all reasonable efforts to provide current and accurate information for the readers of this book. The author and its associates will not be held liable for any unintentional errors or omissions that may be found.

The material in the book may include information by third-parties. Third-party materials comprise of opinions expressed by their owners. As such, the author of this book does not assume responsibility or liability for any third-party material or opinions.

The publication of third-party material does not constitute the author's guarantee of any information, products, services, or opinions contained within third-party material. Use of third-party material does not guarantee that your results will mirror our results. Publication of such third-party material is simply a recommendation and expression of the author's own opinion of that material.

Whether because of the progression of the Internet, or the unforeseen changes in company policy and editorial submission guidelines, what is stated as fact at the time of this writing may become outdated or inapplicable later.

This book is copyright © 2019 by **Cameron Lambert** with all rights reserved. It is illegal to redistribute, copy, or create derivative works from this book whole or in parts. No parts of this report may be reproduced or retransmitted in any forms whatsoever without the written expressed and signed permission from the author.